Sugar-Free Treats (not just) for Kids

Healthy, Easy, Fast & Delicious
Recipes to Make With Your Kids

Nela Kovacovic

Photography by Ashley Despres

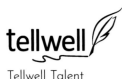

tellwell

Tellwell Talent
www.tellwell.ca

ISBN
978-0-2288-3812-8 (Paperback)
978-0-2288-3814-2 (eBook)

Thanks to all our friends who loved our sugar-free treats and encouraged me to share them with the world. And special thanks to my little kitchen helpers, Ariana, Arwen and Alex, for equally helping and eating the treats.

Table of Contents

Chocolate Obsession

(N)Ice Cream & Popsicles

Introduction

Congratulations! You are an amazing mom! You cared enough to invest money and time into this cookbook. Whether you are a mom who is making conscious healthy food choices and is looking for new recipes, or a mom who is interested in learning healthy alternatives—or perhaps you are a mom-to-be, or a grandma or a mom to fur babies—whatever kind of mom you are, let me tell you that YOU ARE DOING AN AMAZING JOB! Why am I starting with this? Because mom guilt is a real thing and it makes me question myself ALL. THE. FREAKING. TIME.

Yes, this book is about sugar-free baking with your kids and includes some great tips on how to lead a healthier life style, BUT it is definitely NOT about shaming you or making you feel like a crappy mom if you are not 100% giving your kids sugar-free, gluten-free, organic food.

I wrote this book to share with you our family's favorite healthy recipes that are simple, fast and easy to make with your little ones, so you can feel good about what treats you are feeding your family (and yourself)! Maybe you'll learn a thing or two about healthy nutrition along the way, because when we know better, we do better. Let's get real, though: there is no such a thing as a perfect sugar-free diet for kids, because a) it's not realistic, and b) life is about moderation.

I was always interested in a healthy lifestyle. When I had my first baby, I was so worried that I wasn't feeding her "right," that I wasn't giving her enough nutrients and that I would ruin her for the rest of her life (aka: mom guilt). At that time, I joined an online group for moms that proclaimed to be about healthy eating for kids. Sadly, the group quickly turned into a bunch of moms shaming each other for feeding their kids sugar on occasion, not always making food from scratch or, God forbid, giving them store-bought snacks. So, I left as quickly as I joined because that was not the type of mom I aspired to be.

So, why do I care about this sugar-free baking so much? You might say, "What is wrong with having a sugary treat if you don't eat sugar all the time?" I agree—there is absolutely nothing wrong with that—but I see an opportunity to influence and teach our kids lessons that will impact them for life. You know the old adage, "You can't teach an old dog new tricks" (like my husband, although I keep trying), so teach where it counts. I want our kids to know how real, unprocessed food tastes. My hope is that our kids will grow up knowing the benefits of eating healthy food and have the nutritional knowledge that many adults lack. It's about teaching them healthier habits so they start engaging in them organically.

I don't believe kids (or adults) should be deprived of anything (like a treat), but why can't we all enjoy treats that are actually good for us? Let's have our cake and eat it, too!

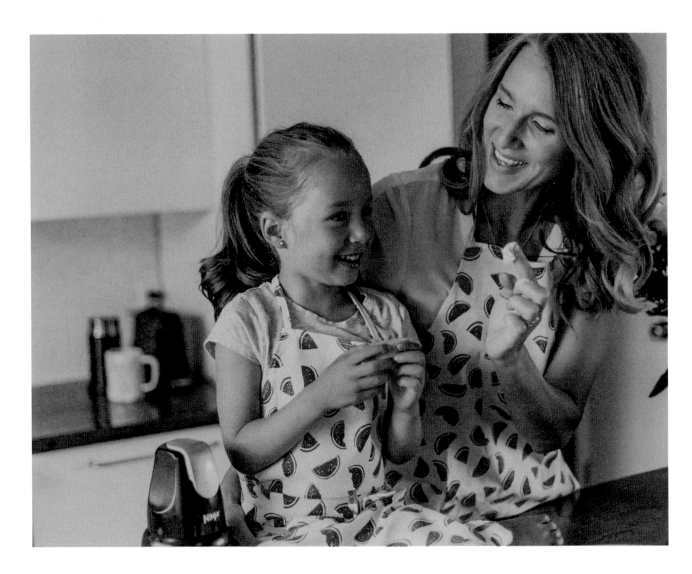

Before we start, please let me share my story with you. It is a classic fairy tale. I know what you're thinking, "Here she goes . . ." Please keep reading. I promise not to disappoint!

I'm originally from a small country—locally referred to as "the heart of Europe"—called Slovakia. After several miscarriages and having lost hope of having kids, my mom finally became pregnant with me. I was born and was told to be a miracle baby.

When I was 11, my mom tragically passed of lung cancer. My dad remarried a lady with an ice-cold heart who hated her new stepchild (told ya—classic fairy tale!). Just like in Cinderella's story, there was nothing I could do to please my stepmom, so when I was of legal age, I packed one bag with my belongings, including a small box of my mom's jewelry, left the house and never looked back.

This is more of a modern fairy tale, as unlike Cinderella, I didn't depend on Prince Charming to save me. Instead, I finished university with a master's degree in TV & Movie Production at the Academy of Performing Arts and commenced a career in national television as a production manager. A few years later, I transitioned into event production, and yes, you guessed it, found

my prince charming. We moved to Canada to experience the amazing country of maple syrup, got married and had three perfect children: Ariana, Arwen and Alex.

Let's back up a bit, though . . . When my husband (boyfriend at that time) suggested we move to Canada, I was NOT on board. I may have used words like "over my dead body" and "no way am I leaving my well-established career to go work at Starbucks." But, after thinking about it and letting it sink in, it really was the perfect time to go see a different country, meet new people and learn a new language.

After arriving in Canada, I started to look for work and quickly realized how difficult this endeavor was with no previous Canadian work experience and thick Slovak-accented English. So, I applied for an "event assistant" position with minimum wage just to get my foot in the door. I had friends telling me that I was crazy to be applying for a position in which I would be underpaid and overqualified. Despite this, I trusted my skills and my experience. I wanted to stay working in my field of expertise—the event industry—so I didn't mind starting small in a new country. I took the job, and after two weeks, I was promoted to the event manager role, planning a tour of corporate outdoor events all over the province. I'm grateful for my former employers Arlene and Brent, who took a chance on me and never treated me like an immigrant. It was very important to believe in myself, not allow my insecurities to get in my way and work hard to achieve my goals.

It's never easy to raise three small children in a country where you have no family or support. I know there are many of you dealing with similar circumstances. As much as I would love a "grandma break" at times, I try to stay grateful for what I have. I believe this chosen path has brought my husband and me closer as friends and as a family unit. Moving across the ocean to a country where we barely knew anyone has been a life-changing experience. Yes, there are times where I feel homesick, miss my friends and wish I had some help with the kids, but I also know that I've gained so much! We've been lucky to make loyal friends who are here for us. I've found a supportive work community, had the opportunity to work on a number of amazing events, won an international event award, become a local event association president and launched my own business. All of this in just eight years and three babies later—thanks to my dedication to working hard and the support of my husband, my friends, and my mom watching over me from wherever she may be.

I would also like to mention my two half-sisters. I realize that makes me sound even more like Cinderella, but my sisters, who are older than me, are from my dad's first marriage before my mom,

and they've always been so supportive of me! I'm grateful to have them in my life. My oldest sister found her home in Israel and my middle sister still lives in Slovakia. Between the three of us and my three cousins, we live in five different countries (Canada, Israel, United Kingdom, Germany and Slovakia). Talk about a multi-cultural bunch! (Spoiler alert: **Sugar-Free Treats from around the Globe** is coming next!)

Now, onto something more relevant to this book. Here are a few things I remember about my mom that shaped me into the person I am today and inspired me to write this cookbook:

1. Her success: She had a great career and it empowered me my whole life that I can do anything . . . even write a cookbook that I'm so passionate about! I hope I can be the same example for my kids and gift them the empowerment to become whatever they want to be!

2. Her love for physical activities: She loved exercising, swimming, skiing . . . She once took me with her to her aerobic classes that were just beginning to gain popularity in our country and I was mind-blown! She loved saunas and taught me to always submerge myself in freezing water afterwards for the health benefits! She loved hiking, and I remember the one time we thought a bear was chasing us (turned out to be a friend who pretended to be a bear—yes, very funny). Exercising is very important for us and is

something I try to teach by example to my kids daily. Whether it is an actual workout, yoga, biking or jumping on a trampoline, we make sure we move our bodies. Not to be skinny and fit into our tightest jeans, but to be healthy and strong!

3. Her love for cooking and healthy eating: My mom loved to pick fresh mushrooms in the mountains and I treasure the memory of her teaching me how to clean them. She would also pick different herbs, dry them and then use them for tea. My father went through a phase of vegetarianism, so we ate a variety of different meals made from soy or other plant-based alternatives. Although I'm not a vegetarian and I strongly believe in food variety (especially if the food comes from a sustainable source), I'm grateful I learned to appreciate plant-based food and limit meat consumption. Thanks to my mom, I was fortune to develop a complex palate and learn about healthy eating from a very young age.

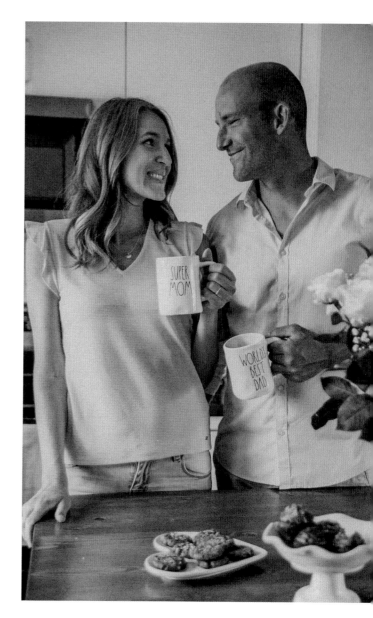

I strongly believe that what you learn as a child impacts you for rest of your life. That is why I am teaching my kids the fundamentals of healthy habits for their future. Whether it's believing in themselves and having the mental strength and discipline to follow their dreams, or moving their bodies to be stronger every day, or fueling their bodies to be the healthiest version of themselves, I hope I can be as good of an example to my kids as my mom was to me.

Why Sugar-Free Treats?

Let's cover the basics. Why is sugar the "enemy"?

Sugar is an empty calorie. Adding it to foods and drinks significantly increases their calorie content without adding any nutritional benefit. The body digests these foods and drinks quickly, spiking blood sugar levels, leading to mood swings, fatigue, headaches and cravings for more sugar without any source of energy.

Too much sugar in kids (or adults) can cause hyperactivity, increase the risk for heart disease, obesity and type 2 diabetes. Sugar interferes with immune functions by feeding bacteria and yeast. Like drugs, sugar floods the brain with dopamine, a feel-good chemical, thus interfering with normal functioning of the brain (aka the sugar rush).

The World Health Organization recommends reducing the intake of sugars in both adults and children to less than 10% of total energy intake.[1] The American Heart Association (AHA) recommends that daily added-sugar intake in kids should not exceed six teaspoons.[2]

Unfortunately, collected data showed that the average North American child consumes 20 to 25 teaspoons of sugar every day! These are crazy numbers that are easily achievable due to our food production. Added sugars hide in many foods including processed frozen foods, cereals, granola, instant oatmeal, salad dressings, ketchup, barbecue sauces, pasta sauces, flavored yogurt, protein bars, and more. It's estimated that 60 - 75 percent of all foods in the supermarket have sugar added to them.

Sugar goes by a lot of different names—more than 50, if we're inspecting nutrition labels. Here are a few to look out for: dextrose, maltose, barley malt, brown sugar, corn sweetener, corn syrup, rice syrup, fructose sweetener, fruit juice concentrates, glucose, high-fructose corn syrup, evaporated cane juice, invert sugar, lactose, malt syrup, molasses, pancake syrup, raw sugar, sucrose, trehalose, and turbinado sugar. To identify an added sugar, be suspicious of words that end with "-ose," as well as names that contain "syrup" or "malt."

But what about products that naturally contain sugar, like fruit and dairy products? By consuming whole foods with naturally occurring sugars, your body digests these foods slowly and the sugar in them offers a steady supply of energy to your

---

[1] "Guideline: Sugars intake for adults and children" (Geneva: World Health Organization, 2015)

[2] "Sugar and Our Children," American Heart Association, accessed October 19, 2019, https://www.yourethecure.org/sugar-and-our-children/.

cells. Yes, they contain the same calories, but they also contain other nutrients, like fiber and a range of vitamins and minerals that support our health and vitality.

There are many people who cut sugar completely, including naturally occurring sugar, but I personally believe the sugars found in fruit are a part of a balanced healthy diet, especially for children.

So how can we decrease sugar intake? I recommend these three simple steps:

1. Say Goodbye to Soda/Pop and Juice

This may not be a surprise for you, but sugary drinks are the single largest source of added sugar in a child's diet. By cutting sweetened drinks out of your kids' diet, you are able to cut over half of their sugar intake! Yes, soda/pop is obvious, but fruit juice is just as bad. Fruit juice is most easily mistaken by parents as a healthy choice. If you buy the natural kind with no added sugar, how could it be wrong? The problem is that because it is in liquid form, it's easy to overconsume. A single glass of apple juice contains the same amount of sugar as three or four apples (without any of the fiber). Your child would never eat four apples at once but drinks a glass of juice in seconds! You see what I mean.

Water is everything (sorry to be so dramatic, but this one is just too close to my heart). Small children, especially, don't need to be drinking juice. You want them to get used to drinking water all the time and then introduce juice as a treat. I'm not a crazy mom who slaps juice out of my kids' hands, but we never have juice at home and my kids enjoy juice as a special treat at birthday parties and other outings. Don't get me wrong: if my kids see juice, they'll ask for it, but they usually drink one glass for the novelty and then ask for water when thirsty. If your kids get used to the taste of juice at a young age, they'll have a harder time accepting to drink plain water. This will result in teenagers and adults fighting the common soda addiction. Teach your kids to drink water and EAT fruit. By eating whole fruit, they'll get extra vitamins and fiber. Fiber is important for our digestive health and regular bowel movements. Fiber also helps us feel fuller for longer and can improve cholesterol and blood sugar levels.

If your kids are not big on water (yet), start with making fruit-infused flavored water. Turn plain water into something beautiful, refreshing and naturally colorful by adding some frozen fruit, herbs (like mint), lemon or lime juice and ice. We especially love adding these in summer months to make our water more fun and refreshing. My kids mix various concoctions by themselves and are proud to make their own special fancy drinks!

2. Make Homemade Treats

This may looks like I'm building a case for success for this cookbook, and yes, partially I am, but more important, by making homemade treats, you are in charge of what your kids eat. A large part of kids' daily sugar intake is hidden inside various packaged and processed foods, many of which are disguised and marketed as healthy. The number one reason processed food has so much added sugar is to act as a preservative, extend shelf life, and make the foods more appetizing. In recent years, the public has become increasingly aware of the negative side effects of added sugar, leading to food companies getting creative with their product labeling. I'll talk about this further in the book, but the bottom line is that if you make your own treats, you know exactly what is in them. That is why all my recipes only use whole food simple ingredients. Involving your kids in the process will enable them to identify these whole foods in their natural form.

Yes, an occasional treat won't kill your kids, and I'm not suggesting you should be perfect and never feed your kids anything store-bought. But why not teach your kids to appreciate the taste of food without added sugars and preservatives? Making sugar-free treats will satisfy their cravings and you can feel good about what you are feeding them.

Additionally, baking together is a fun, family-bonding activity. It's like doing crafts, but with a yummy treat at the end. Baking helps your children to develop fine motor skills, eye-hand coordination, and even early concepts of math and science. They are also more likely to enjoy a meal they helped make. It takes some patience letting your kids "help" you (and will likely mean a bigger mess), but to see your kids excited about the healthy treat they made is definitely worth it!

3. Fat vs Sugar

Don't freak out; I'm not going to suggest that you serve your kids bacon at each meal. The idea of accepting fat as being "healthy" was very difficult for me, personally, as I was always taught that fat is bad. It is important to know that not all fats are unhealthy and that many foods that are touted as "low-fat" may do more harm than good when it comes to your kids' overall health.

One of the biggest contradictions is that these "low-fat" foods are usually pumped full of preservatives, additives, and extra sugar to boost flavor and enhance taste. On the other hand, unsaturated fatty acids found in foods like avocados, olive oil and nuts boost heart health, lower cholesterol levels, and alleviate inflammation. Saturated fatty acids such as coconut oil have also been linked to better brain function. When our children consume a meal that contains healthy fat, they're less likely to feel hungry soon after the meal as healthy fats help regulate blood sugar levels. So, if you have to choose between full-fat plain yogurt (the taste comes from its creaminess) or low-fat flavored yogurt (the taste comes from a ton of sugar), the choice is pretty simple.

So, which fats are good for us and our kids? Refined vegetable oils, processed meats and snack foods like chips, crackers and baked goods are generally high in disease-causing, artery-clogging trans fats that should be avoided at all costs. Trans fats are not found in nature. They are a by-product of the process that turns healthy oils into solid fats, such as margarine, and prevents baked goods from going rancid. The key to finding healthy fats is to look for ingredients that are unprocessed and natural such as avocados, nuts, seeds, eggs, fatty fish and dark chocolate (yay for chocolate making it on the list!).

Choosing an overall balanced diet is key, and healthy fats should definitely be a part of your menu.

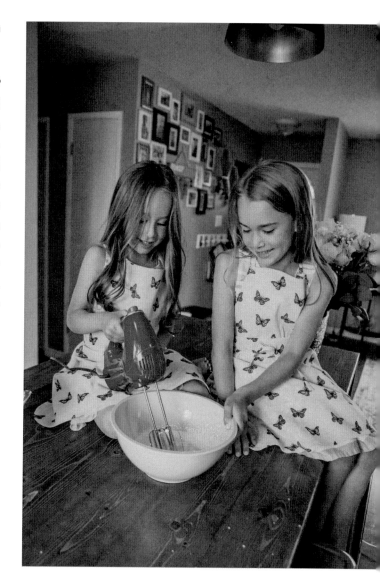

Simple rules I follow:

1. Read labels

Sugar is hidden in many foods—even ones that don't taste sweet. Make sure to check the labels of packaged or processed foods. Products with health claims such as "diet," "natural" or "low-fat" may still be loaded with sugar. Make sure you read both the nutritional value and ingredient list, as some products may contain naturally occurring sugar, which is okay. Ingredients are listed by weight on packaged foods, with the main ingredients listed first. The more of one item, the higher up on the list it appears.

There are a few tricks to watch out for: food manufacturers try to trick you into making their products appear healthier. Often, they list smaller amounts of three or four types of sugar in a single product. These sugars then appear further down on the ingredient list, making a product seem low in sugar—when, in sum, sugar is one of its main ingredients.

Another issue is portion size. Food companies often reduce the portion size to make products appear lower in sugar. If you are comparing two different products to check witch one has less sugar, make sure to check portion size, as the one with a lower sugar amount may actually have more sugar overall.

2. Drink water

Yup. You've heard it and I'm saying it again!! You and your kids don't need anything but water to drink (okay, you as a mom, may also need coffee and wine for survival, but that doesn't count). Read labels for loose teas, as well, as many contain—you guessed it!—added sugar.

3. No "kids' food"

My European heritage always kicks in when we get to the restaurant. It drives me crazy that a really great restaurant with a gourmet menu offers the same five choices for children: pizza, pasta, mac and cheese, fish fingers and chicken nuggets. Why is it assumed that kids only eat these five meals? Yes, we definitely eat pizza, but we go to a pizza place and enjoy pizza as a family. There is no such a thing as "kids' food" in our household.

First of all, I refuse to make something different for them than what I'm serving; what I cook is what everyone will eat (sorry, not sorry). Second, why would I serve my kids something I don't want to eat? This rule was established as soon as our kids started eating solid foods. Of course I would not season their salmon as much as ours, but they were served and ate the same meal. I love the quote from Pamela Druckerman's book **Bringing Up Bébé**: "Treat your child like a little gourmet, and they will (gradually) rise to the occasion." (If you are not familiar with this book, I highly recommend it. For any new mom-to-be, it is the only parenting book you need.)

4. Don't buy it

Simple as that! If we don't have it, they can't get it. My husband, Andy, says I'm not strict enough with our children, and that may be true to some extent. He figures if we had a bunch of chocolate, candies and cookies at home, I would have a hard time saying no to my kids (or to myself for that matter). So, if it's not in our house, we are not having it and we are forced to whip something up quickly that satisfies our cravings—hence, how all the recipes in this cookbook were created!

5. Lead by example

It would probably not work if I offered my kids a plate with raw veggies, while I munched on fries. If my kids see me eating healthy, they don't actually see me eating "healthy." They see me eating, and what I eat is the norm for them. Vegetables or fruit are always part of a meal without talking about it. As a study from Stanford University has shown, children learn a lot from the eating habits of their parents. They tend to copy their parents' food choices in the long run.[3]

6. Don't obsess about it

It's a funny thing but kids can feel when something really matters to us and that's usually the time when they decide to act up. You know, like that one time you really don't want to be late and they decide to have a meltdown because they can't find their favorite shoes (meanwhile they are already wearing their favorite shoes, but they claim those are NOT their favorite). I've found that if I obsess about my kids eating too much of this and not enough of that then that's the time they intentionally don't cooperate.

Negative attention is attention, so if you put energy into it—so will they! Our rule is to be casual about it. We try to explain the importance of our food choices, but don't obsess about it. Meals are a time for the whole family to be together and enjoy one another's company and not fight about food.

7. Moderation

Life is about moderation. Yes, I try to make homemade popsicles to enjoy on a hot sunny day at home, but we also go out for a bike ride and buy ice cream. Yes, I bake healthy sugar-free desserts, but when we go out to eat at a restaurant, we order regular dessert. When at a birthday party, we enjoy birthday cake or cupcakes. Let your kids have a treat on occasion, but keep portions in mind. Coming from Europe, I was shocked by the portions in North America. You can have your cake and eat it, too—but you don't need half of an entire cake just for yourself! Lastly, don't feel guilty while enjoying a treat because—you know it—life is about moderation!

---

[3]   Maya Adam, MD. "Child Nutrition and Cooking." (Stanford School of Medicine, 2020)

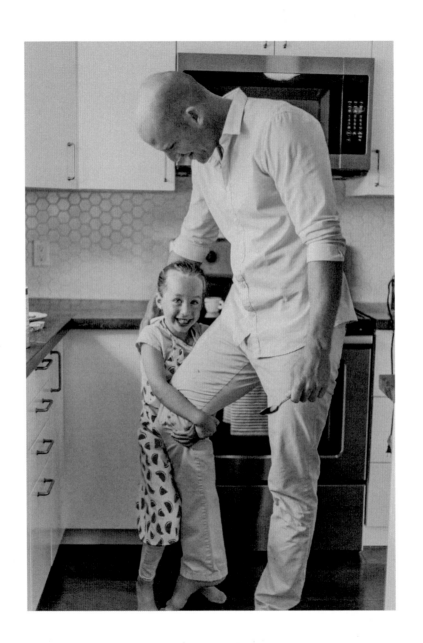

Quick Recipe Notes

You will notice that most of my recipes use similar ingredients. These are what I consider to be "staples." I'm all about quick and easy. I don't like to buy a specific ingredient just for one recipe and then never use it again. I like to have on hand most of the ingredients I regularly use with alternation, if needed. I also like to limit the ingredient list to a minimum. Less is more. Also, who has time!? The recipes are quick and should take no more than 15 to 20 minutes to make (max 30 minutes if you have your toddler "helping" you).

The following ingredients are repeated in many recipes:

Nuts and seeds—raw, natural, unsalted: Mounting evidence suggests that eating nuts and seeds daily can lower your risk of diabetes and heart disease and may even lengthen your life.[4] Nuts are loaded with antioxidants, including the polyphenols that can combat oxidative stress by neutralizing free radicals—unstable molecules that may cause cell damage and increase disease risk. Walnuts, chia seeds and hemp seeds are really high in omega-3 fatty acids, which support your brain health and help reduce inflammation. I recommend storing nuts and seeds in the freezer and using a variety to get nutritional benefits from the different types.

Nut or seed butter—natural without added sugar: As an alternative to fresh nuts and seeds, I use nut or seed butter in many recipes. Nut and seed butter contains natural healthy fats that are good for your heart and cholesterol. They are a phenomenal source of vitamins, minerals and nutrients. All nut butters contain heart-healthy unsaturated fats, phytosterols, protein and fiber. Healthy, high-quality nut butters are made without additional sweeteners or preservatives. Be sure to check the label for these extra ingredients and also beware of the varieties that contain hydrogenated oil, as these contain unwanted trans fats. Manufacturers add these ingredients to keep the oil from separating during storage; however, this separation is normal and just requires that you stir the seed or nut butter before using it. To keep the nut-butter oil from separating, store the jars upside down in your pantry.

My preferred butter to use in most of my recipes is peanut butter or almond butter, but you can use any nut or seed butter of your choice depending on allergies and taste.

---

4   "Eating Nuts May Reduce Cardiovascular Disease," American Heart Association, accessed March 21, 2019, https://newsroom.heart.org/news/eating-nuts-may-reduce-cardiovascular-disease-risk-for-people-with-diabetes/.

Fresh fruit: Fruit is an excellent source of essential vitamins and minerals, and it is high in fiber. Fruit also contains a wide range of health-boosting antioxidants and is a natural sweetener. I recommend eating fresh fruit that is in season and didn't have to travel a thousand miles to get to you. Get it as local as possible, preferably grown right in your garden or bought from a farmer's market. However, since that is not always an option, buy organic fruit from grocery stores when possible. As that may get expensive, the second best option is to buy frozen fruit.

Frozen fruit: The number one benefit of frozen fruit is that fruit is picked and frozen at peak ripeness. Frozen fruit retains a comparable— or higher—vitamin, mineral and phytochemical content to its fresh counterpart. Fresh produce can lose nutritional value the longer it sits out past its harvest date, due to enzymatic activity and oxidation. When fresh fruit is not in season, frozen fruit is often a cheaper and healthier alternative.

Dried fruit—without added sweetener: Dried fruit is tasty and delicious but it is also rich in minerals, proteins, fiber and vitamins. Make sure you read labels and avoid dry fruit with added sugar. Some dried fruit is coated with sugar and syrup before drying to make it sweeter. For example, most dried cranberries have added sugar. Some dried fruit has added juice instead of sugar, which is a healthier alternative but still not ideal. The dried fruit I use in my recipes mostly includes dates, raisins, prunes, goji berries and shredded coconut. Dates are the best natural sweetener and are also referred to as the "candy" of nature. They are naturally sweet but contain vitamins and minerals that are good for our bodies. They, along with most dried fruit, are high in calories and should be eaten in moderation. If you are not familiar with goji berries, I suggest you look into them. They are called a superfood due to their nutritional value, and I love adding them to our oatmeal or baking as an alternative to raisins.

Oats: I avoid using flour in all my recipes. I believe in whole food ingredients that are not processed (or minimally processed), and that is why I opt to use oats as a substitute in many traditional flour recipes. Oats have amazing health benefits, including lowering cholesterol and stabilizing blood glucose levels. They are also loaded with soluble fiber, which slows digestion and keeps us full for a longer time, helping us maintain steady energy levels. Oats make a great gluten-free alternative, but be sure to use certified gluten-free oats. Without the certification, the oats may have been cross-contaminated with gluten-containing grains at some point in their production.

Eggs—organic, pastured (free-range), or best right from a farm: I know they are more expensive, but the health and environmental benefits are worth it. If you are vegan, for most of the recipes that are not already vegan, you can substitute the eggs with finely ground flaxseed.

Here is how: mix 1 tablespoon flaxseed meal (ground flaxseed) with 3 tablespoons water and add to the recipe instead of 1 egg.

Maple syrup: The only sweetener other than fruit I like to use. You will find in a few recipes I suggest adding maple syrup. It is always optional and all my recipes work without it. If you have a toddler, I strongly recommend you avoid using any sweetener. If you have older kids who are used to eating sugary treats, you can always add more maple syrup so their taste buds are able to slowly adjust. These recipes have so many great wholesome ingredients that even if there is added maple syrup, they still have many nutritional benefits in comparison to regular store-bought baked goods that are loaded with sugar and trans fats. Maple syrup is high in antioxidants and rich in minerals, including calcium, potassium, iron, zinc and manganese. However, like other natural sweeteners, maple syrup is high in calories and should be consumed in moderation. If you prefer a different kind of sweetener, go for it, but I find organic maple syrup works best for us.

Chocolate chips: For some of my recipes, I suggest adding chocolate cut into chunks or chocolate chips. I recommend using dark chocolate when possible; the higher cacao it contains equals more good fat and less added sugar. Quality dark chocolate is rich in fiber, iron, magnesium, copper, manganese and a few other minerals. Look for dairy-free chocolate to keep the recipes dairy-free and vegan.

Coconut Cream: I like using coconut cream as a plant based alternative to whipping cream. To get a heavy coconut cream, place canned coconut milk in the refrigerator overnight (I usually store it in the fridge to have on hand when needed). This will make the milk fat separate and solidify on top. Open the can and scoop out the heavy white coconut cream from top. You will be left with clear water on the bottom of the can. Depending on the brand you are using, some cans will have more cream and less water. You can use the coconut water as a substitution for almond milk when making smoothies or popsicles—or pour the water into an ice cube mold and use the coconut ice cubes in flavored water (or your favorite vodka cocktail!).

Spices: The following are the most commonly used in my recipes to add flavor and I recommend having them on hand in your pantry: vanilla extract, ground cinnamon powder and raw 100% cocoa powder.

Pinch of salt: For the longest time, I would ignore the call for a "pinch of salt" in sweet recipes until I came across an article explaining that adding bit of salt to baking will actually bring the sweet taste out.[5] Salt enhances and intensifies food's other flavors. Go figure! Seeing as we are mainly working with whole food ingredients, we definitely want all the flavors to come out!

Recipes Terms:

Sugar-free – without added sweetener. Many recipes online are called sugar free because they don't have any refined sugar, but they have number of added sweeteners so they are not truly sugar free. I wanted to go further and give you true sugar free recipes without ANY added sweetener other than fruits. I'm very proud to say that majority of my recipes are 100% sugar free!

Gluten-free – does not contain gluten. Since I don't add any flour to my recipes, they are all gluten-free. The only base ingredient I work with is oats. Oats are naturally gluten free, but as some oats are often processed in the same facilities as gluten-containing grains, they may not be safe for people with gluten allergies. That's why I recommend getting certified gluten free oats, to ensure they are not contaminated and safe for everyone.

Dairy-free – does not contain dairy. To make most of my recipes dairy-free, you have the option of using the milk of your choice. We prefer unsweetened almond milk. When using chocolate chips, make sure to purchase the dairy-free chocolate.

Vegan – without the use of any animal products. My sister and her whole family are vegan, so I made them test my recipes with vegan substitutions to make sure they worked and tasted delicious. As mentioned before, I like using fresh organic pastured eggs, but if you are vegan, the flaxseed substitution should work for most of the recipes.

Nut-free – does not contain nuts. Many of my recipes include nuts as we are a bit nutty - huge nut fans! For each category, I made sure to include at least a few nut free recipes and/or substitutions.

Raw – Recipes that don't need to be baked or cooked.

---

5   "Make Perfect Porridge," Jamie Oliver, accessed on March 29, 2019, https://www.jamieoliver.com/features/make-perfect-porridge/.

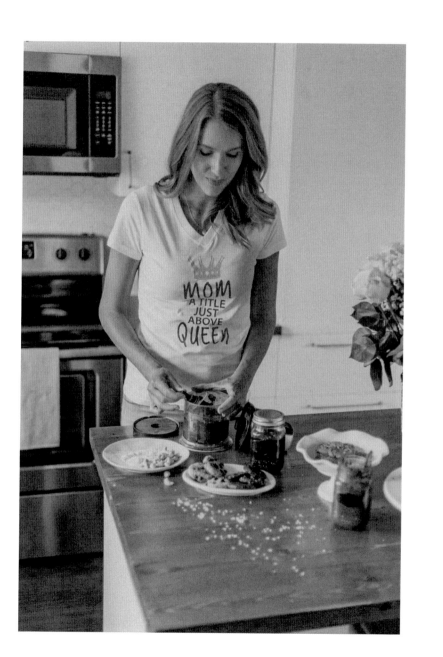

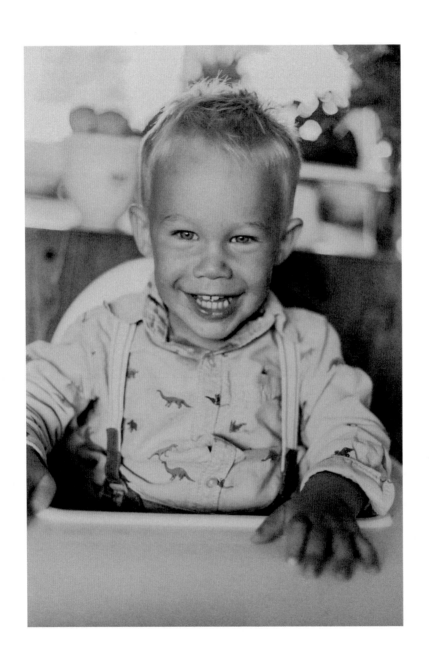

Breakfast

Having a well-balanced breakfast is proven to stabilize energy levels, preventing that mid-morning crash, cut sugar cravings and help eliminate additional snacking. But what is a well-balanced breakfast? Morning cereals are marketed as healthy breakfast options, but did you know that one serving of most cereals contains more sugar than the daily recommended sugar intake? Not to mention how low their nutritional values are, causing energy levels to go up right after finishing eating only to fall rapidly after a few minutes. This spike and fall in energy results in you and your kids feeling tired for rest of the morning. Breakfast with lower sugar content improves short-term memory and attention spans at school. Giving your child a breakfast which contains fiber keeps adrenaline levels constant and makes the school day a more productive experience.

I'm not saying you can never serve cereals again, but make sure to read the labels for what is included in your kids' cereals and how much sugar per serving they have. There are a few brands that now offer cereals made from beans with lower sugar content which are amazing.

I created this section to give you some ideas for healthier breakfast foods. I know that some of these recipes take more time (and no one has time on a school morning!), so I encourage you to make them in advance and store them in the fridge or freezer (waffles, pancakes, granola) or make them on a weekend. In our house, Saturday is our crepes day and our go-to breakfast during the week is Our Signature Breakfast Bowl or Protein Waffles and Banana Pancakes from the freezer.

Our Signature Breakfast Bowl

Sugar-free, Gluten-free, Dairy-free, Vegan, Nut-free

I already talked about the health benefits of oats. Oats keep us full for a long time and maintain steady energy levels. By adding different seeds, fruit and nuts, we are making a healthy breakfast bomb, setting up our bodies and mind for a successful day! This is a very simple recipe that you can modify to satisfy your taste buds. I included three different ways of preparing this recipe. The convenience and time saving benefits of using the microwave on busy mornings is worth it! As some people try to eliminate the usage of microwaves, I included a regular stove-top recipe, too. You can also soak the oats in water or milk of your choice overnight to eliminate cooking altogether.

Ingredients (for two breakfast bowls)

- 1 cup oats (certified gluten-free, as needed; we use organic quick oats)
- 1 & 1/2 cup water (or milk of your choice)
- 1/2 cup nuts (omit for nut-free version; I love to mix in walnuts and pecans)
- 1 cup fresh fruit (any fruit of your liking)

- 2 tablespoons unsweetened dried fruit (we love goji berries or raisins)
- 2 tablespoons seeds (chia, hempseeds, sunflower seeds)
- 1 teaspoon cinnamon or cocoa powder (optional)
- Pinch of salt

Directions

In microwave: Put all ingredients in a bowl and microwave for about one minute (depending on the type of oats you are using the time may be longer). You may want to experiment with how much liquid you use and how long you are warming them for, as every microwave is a bit different. Stir before serving.

On stove top: In a small saucepan, combine the oats with water or milk of your choice. Bring to a boil, then reduce heat to low and simmer until the liquid has been absorbed (around 5-10 minutes). Stir occasionally to prevent oats from sticking to the bottom of the pan. Pour into bowl and mix in the remaining ingredients.

Overnight: Stir all ingredients together, except for fresh fruit, in an airtight container. Put into the fridge overnight. Take out in the morning and add fresh fruit before serving.

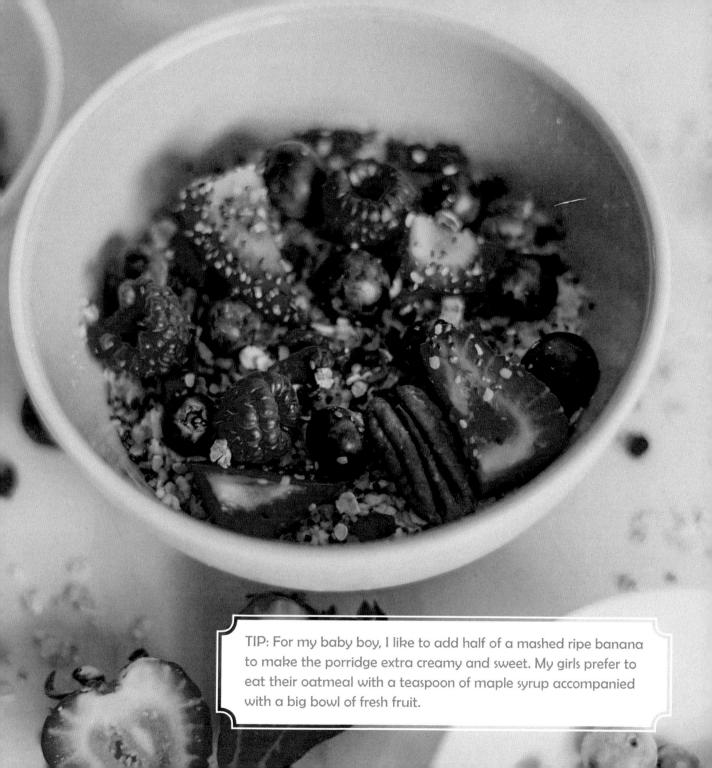

TIP: For my baby boy, I like to add half of a mashed ripe banana to make the porridge extra creamy and sweet. My girls prefer to eat their oatmeal with a teaspoon of maple syrup accompanied with a big bowl of fresh fruit.

Protein Waffles

Sugar-free, Gluten-free, Dairy-free, Nut-free

These waffles are super simple with only 3 main ingredients. They are full of protein without the addition of protein powder, which is not recommended for children. The eggs and cottage cheese give you and your kids all the protein you need.

Ingredients

- 2 cups oats (certified gluten-free, as needed)
- 2 cups cottage cheese
- 6 eggs
- 1/2 teaspoon vanilla extract
- Pinch of salt

Directions

1. Preheat a waffle iron. Use coconut oil (or non-stick spray) for the top and bottom of the waffle iron. I do this after each waffle to make sure my waffles doesn't stick.
2. In a food processor, blend oats until they are fine and begin to look powdery, like flour. Add eggs, cottage cheese, vanilla and salt and blend until smooth.
3. Pour about 1/2 cup of the mixture into the waffle iron, close gently and cook until golden brown and crisp, about 4-5 minutes.

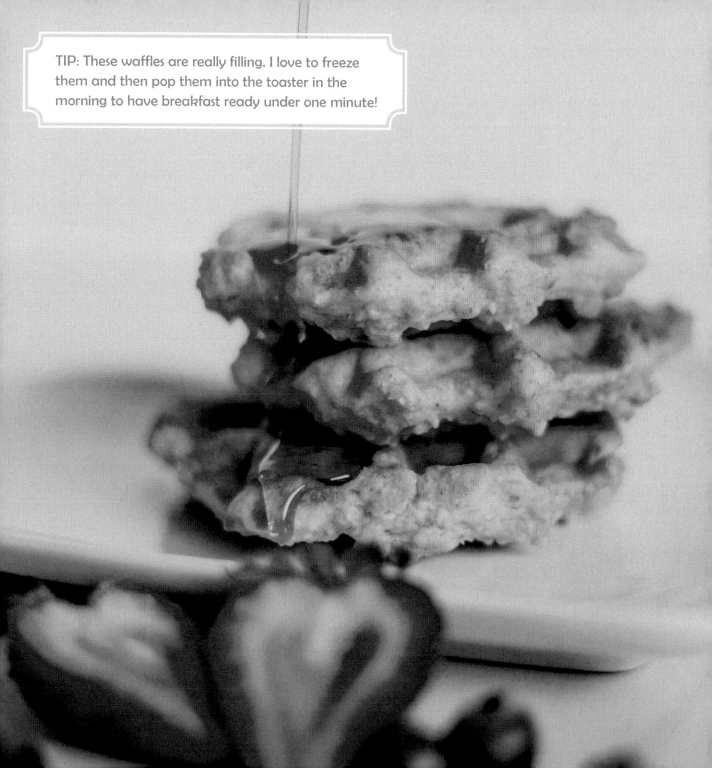

TIP: These waffles are really filling. I love to freeze them and then pop them into the toaster in the morning to have breakfast ready under one minute!

Easy Banana Pancakes

Sugar-free, Gluten-free, Dairy-free, Nut-free

Initially, we were not the biggest fans of pancakes. Both myself and my husband come from Europe, so instead of pancakes, we were used to crepes. Only after moving to Canada and becoming more familiar with local traditions did we discover a love for pancakes. These easy banana pancakes are perfect if you have ripe bananas on hand and are craving a delicious sweet breakfast.

Ingredients

- 1/2 cup oats (certified gluten-free, as needed)
- 2 eggs
- 1 banana
- 1/4 cup apple sauce
- 1 teaspoon vanilla extract
- 1/2 teaspoon cinnamon
- Coconut oil for frying

Directions

1. Blend oats in a food processor until finely ground.
2. Add the rest of the ingredients - eggs, banana, apple sauce, vanilla extract and cinnamon, and blend until fully combined.
3. Heat the oil in a frying pan over medium heat. Spoon one tablespoon of the dough into the pan and repeat to fill the pan, keeping some space enabling you to flip them.
4. Turn the heat to medium/low and allow to cook for around 2-3 minutes per side. Repeat until mixture is used up.

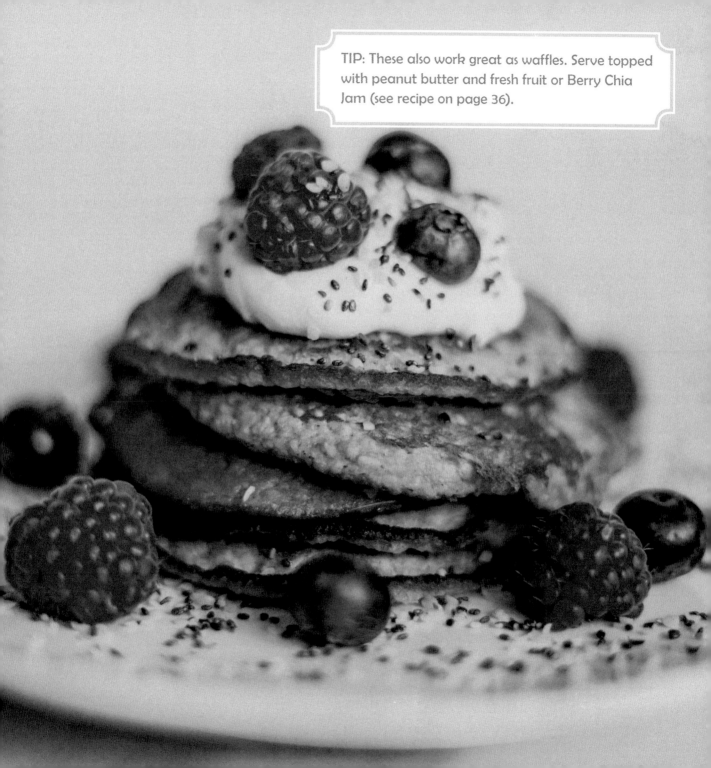

TIP: These also work great as waffles. Serve topped with peanut butter and fresh fruit or Berry Chia Jam (see recipe on page 36).

Healthy Crepes

Sugar-free, Gluten-free, Dairy-free, Nut-free

Crepes are our favorite weekend breakfast meal. It took me a long time to find the best ratio of ingredients to avoid using flour without resulting in the crepes tasting like an omelet or being impossible to flip. By adding the banana, the batter turns out nice and smooth with a hint of sweetness.

Ingredients

- 1 cup oats (certified gluten-free, as needed)
- 2 eggs
- 1 ripe banana
- 1 & 1/2 cup milk of your choice
- Pinch of salt
- Coconut oil for coating pan

Directions

1. Blend oats in a food processor until you achieve a finely ground, flour-like consistency.
2. Add the eggs, banana, milk, salt and blend. The batter should be smooth and not too thick.
3. Heat a lightly oiled non-stick pan or griddle over medium-high heat. Pour the batter onto the pan, using around 1/4 cup for each crepe. With a circular motion, tilt the pan so that the batter coats the bottom of the pan evenly.
4. Cook the crepe for about 2 minutes. Once the bottom is golden brown, flip it. Cook for about 2 more minutes on the other side.
5. Add toppings of your liking, roll and serve.

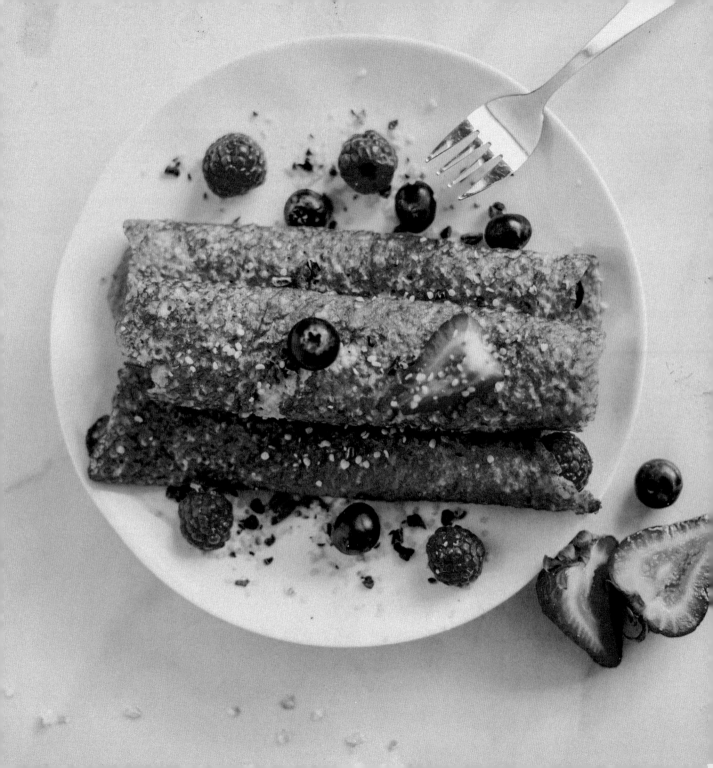

Homemade Granola

Sugar-free, Gluten-free, Dairy-free, Vegan

You may already know this, but most of the store-bought granola that is marketed as healthy is actually full of sugar. It will take you less than 10 minutes to prep your own, and you will have an easy, quick breakfast on hand. You can customize this granola using nuts, seeds and dried fruit of your kids' liking. Below is our favorite combination.

Ingredients

- 2 bananas
- 1/4 cup almond butter (or nut/seed butter of your choice)
- 1/4 cup coconut oil, melted
- 2 cups oats (certified gluten-free, as needed)
- 1 cup chopped nuts (walnuts, pecans, cashews, almond)

- 1/2 cup seeds of your choice (hempseeds, chia seeds, sunflower seeds)
- 1/4 cup raisins (or unsweetened dried fruit of your choice)
- 2 teaspoon cinnamon
- Pinch of salt
- 1 teaspoon 100 % cacao nibs (optional)

Directions

1. Preheat the oven to 300°F/150°C and line a baking tray with parchment paper or a silicone baking sheet.
2. Mash bananas in a large mixing bowl. Add almond butter and melted coconut oil and stir together well to combine. Add oats, chopped nuts, seeds, raisins, cinnamon and salt and stir well until everything is thoroughly combined.
3. Spread onto baking tray. Bake for around 30 minutes. Stir every 10 minutes to get all pieces consistently crunchy.
4. Store in an airtight container for up to 2 weeks.

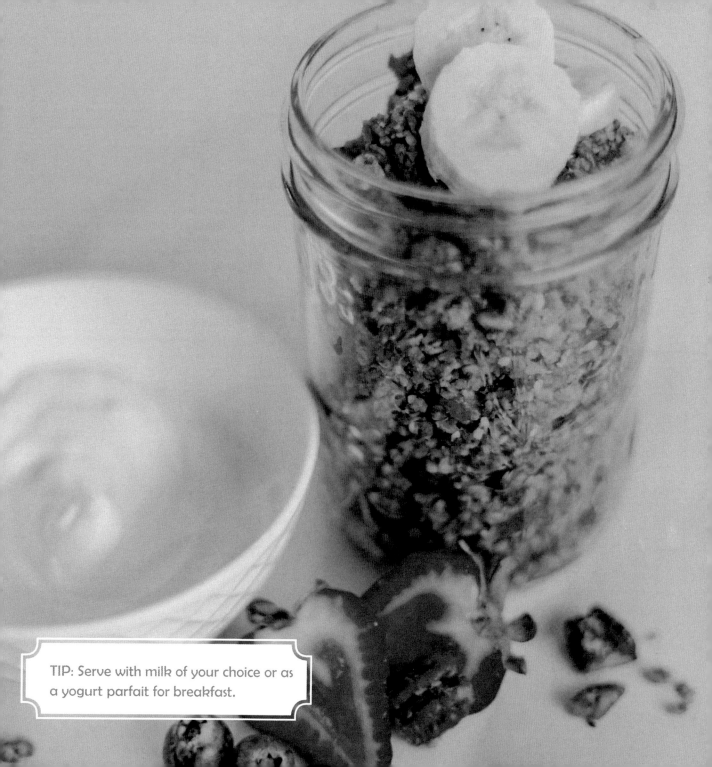

TIP: Serve with milk of your choice or as a yogurt parfait for breakfast.

Protein Breakfast Cups

Sugar-free, Gluten-free, Nut-free, Raw

These protein breakfast cups are a lifesaver for a busy mom! We all have those mornings when we are out the door before putting anything but coffee in our mouths. Dry cottage cheese contains high amounts of natural protein but doesn't have a strong taste (or any taste, for that matter). I invented these cups as my post-workout snack, but they make a great breakfast or a yummy addition to a school lunch box.

Ingredients

- 1 cup dry cottage cheese
- 1 cup unsweetened vanilla yogurt (or natural plain yogurt)
- 1/4 cup applesauce, unsweetened
- 1 teaspoon cinnamon
- 1 teaspoon vanilla extract (omit if using vanilla yogurt)
- 1/4 cup raisins (or dried fruit of your choice)
- 1/4 cup pecans or walnuts (omit for nut-free version)

Directions

1. In a food processor, blend cottage cheese, yogurt, apple sauce and cinnamon.
2. Stir in raisins and nuts. Put double the amount of dried fruit if omitting nuts.
3. Place into cups and refrigerate until ready to eat. Eat within 3 days or freeze for up to 3 months.

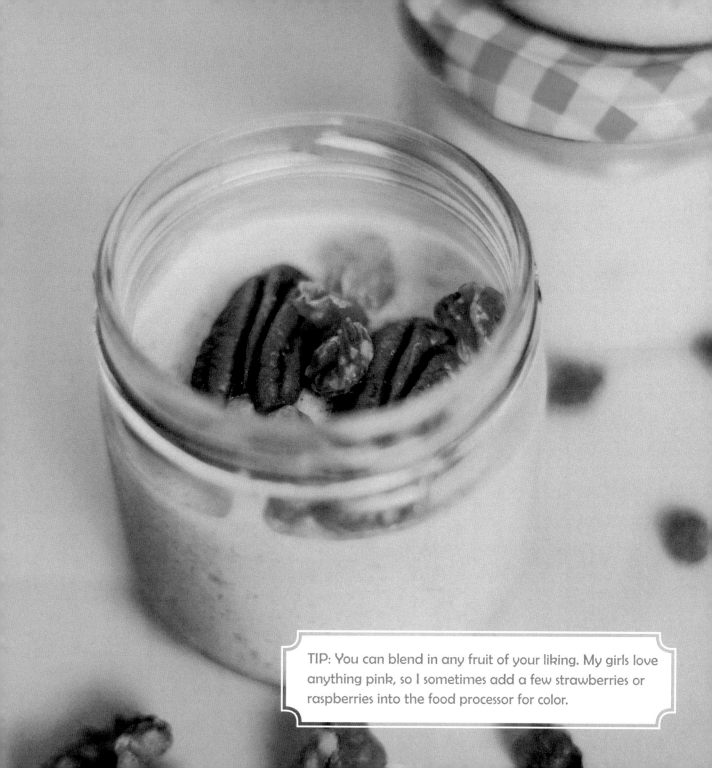

TIP: You can blend in any fruit of your liking. My girls love anything pink, so I sometimes add a few strawberries or raspberries into the food processor for color.

Mango Chia Pudding

Sugar-free, Gluten-free, Dairy-free, Vegan, Nut-free, Raw

Chia pudding is one of the hippest things out there! Chia seeds are rich in fiber, protein, omega-3 fatty acids, antioxidants and micronutrients. We find the chia pudding without any kind of sweetener pretty bland, so adding the pureed mango definitely does the trick!

Ingredients

- 1 cup milk of your choice (I use almond milk)
- 2 tablespoons chia seeds
- 1/2 cup mango

Directions

1. Mix milk and chia seeds in a glass or breakfast bowl and let it soak overnight.
2. When ready to serve, puree mango in a food processor. Stir into the chia pudding, or layer on top and serve.

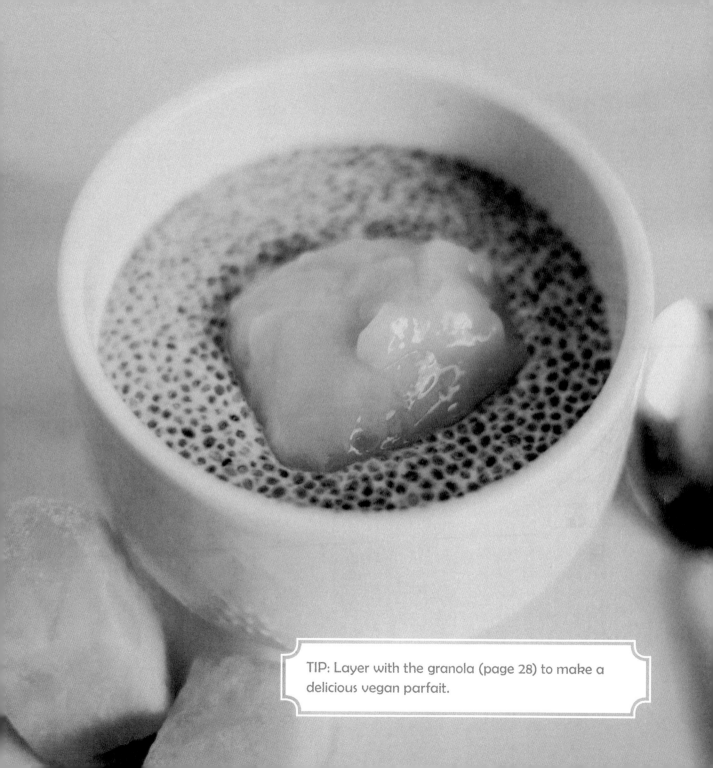

TIP: Layer with the granola (page 28) to make a delicious vegan parfait.

Strawberry Banana Smoothie Bowl

Sugar-free, Gluten-free, Dairy-free, Vegan, Nut-free, Raw

If you are looking for a light breakfast or a quick snack idea, look no further. The smoothie bowl with its add-ons is a bit more filling than a regular smoothie and looks so pretty, too! Since this is a cold breakfast and I prefer for my kids to eat something warm in the morning, I like to make this as a mid-morning snack during hot days.

Ingredients

- 1/2 cup frozen strawberries
- 1 ripe banana
- 1/2 cup milk of your choice (I use almond milk)
- For toppings (any of the following): shredded coconut, chia seeds, hemp seeds, fresh fruit of your choice, cacao nibs or granola (see page 28 for Homemade Granola recipe)

Directions

1. Mix the milk, strawberries and banana in the food processor or blender and process until smooth. Add a little bit of ice if the mixture is not thick enough (it should be a bit thicker than a regular smoothie)
2. Pour into a bowl and add toppings of your choice.
3. Serve immediately.

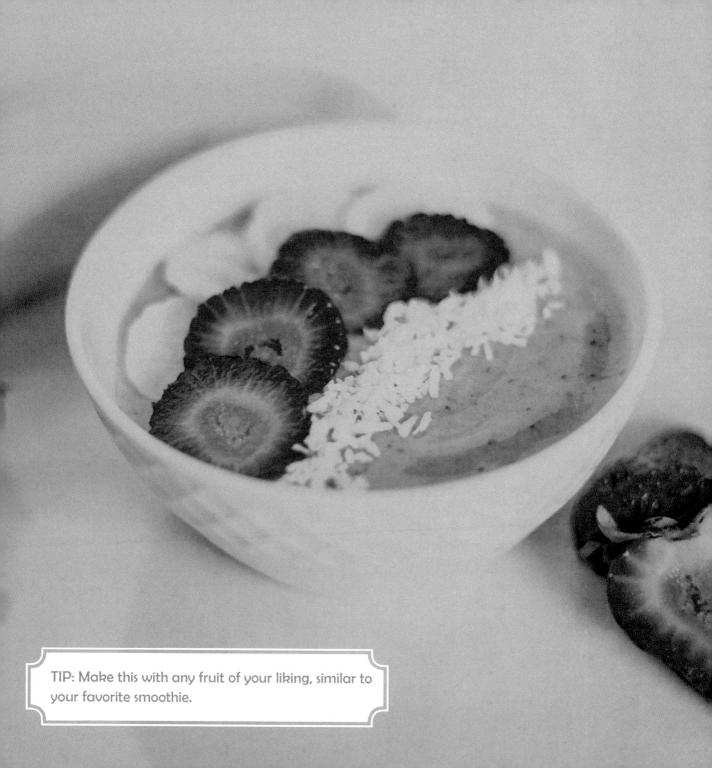

TIP: Make this with any fruit of your liking, similar to your favorite smoothie.

Berry Chia Jam

Gluten-free, Dairy-free, Vegan, Nut-free

This Berry Chia Jam is pure perfection! My kids love everything with jam—waffles, pancakes, crepes, yogurt, peanut-butter sandwiches . . . but I wasn't happy with how much sugar regular jam contains. And every "sugar-free" jam I was able to find actually contains the same or even more artificial sweeteners. This jam has only a hint of maple syrup if you choose to add it, but has no preservatives or any other chemicals. The chia seeds are used to create a "jam" consistency. Chia seeds are an excellent source of omega-3 fatty acids, rich in antioxidants, and they provide fiber, iron and calcium. Win-win-win!

Ingredients

- 3 cups frozen mixed berries of your choice (blueberries, strawberries, raspberries, blackberries, cherries)
- 2 tablespoons maple syrup (optional)
- 2 tablespoons chia seeds

Directions

1. Add frozen mixed berries in a small saucepan and cook over low to medium heat until they start shimmering, about 10 minutes. (Or get distracted with kids, forget what you were doing and come back when the mixture is boiling out of the pot. True story!)
2. Break down the berries with a fork and add maple syrup, if desired.
3. Stir in chia seeds and cook on low for another 5 minutes until the jam thickens.
4. Pour into a glass container and keep sealed in fridge for up to 2 weeks.

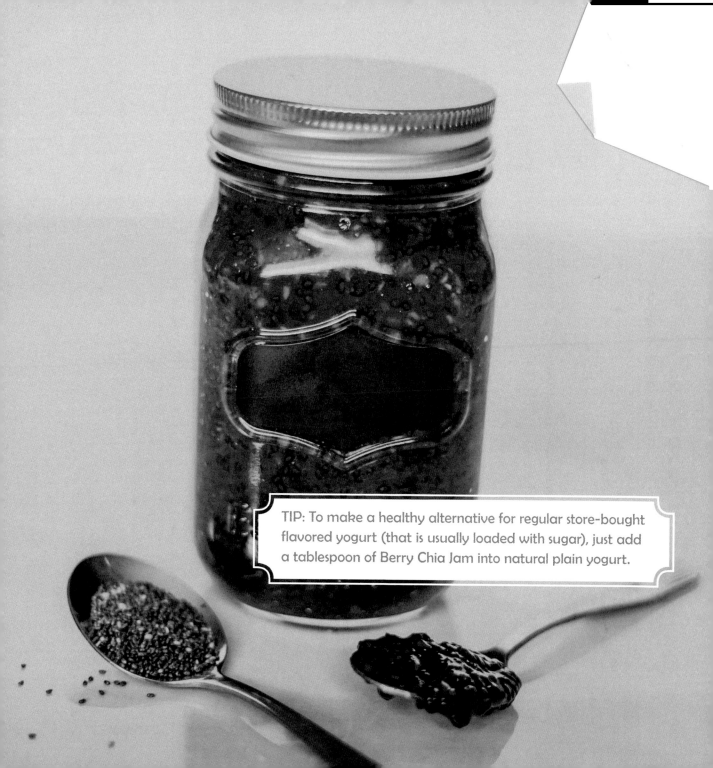

TIP: To make a healthy alternative for regular store-bought flavored yogurt (that is usually loaded with sugar), just add a tablespoon of Berry Chia Jam into natural plain yogurt.

Chocolate Hazelnut Spread

Gluten-free, Dairy-free, Vegan, Raw

I have a thing for store-bought chocolate hazelnut spread. I confess: it's my weakness. I definitely need to follow my own rule "don't buy it," otherwise I'll eat it all in one evening (after the kids are in bed). So, obviously, I had to create my own version without sugar. (Disclaimer: if you are expecting it to taste exactly the same as the store-bought brand, you will be disappointed. But it is as close as it gets and I'd say a pretty good alternative to satisfy your sweet tooth.)

Ingredients

- 2 cups hazelnuts
- 1/2 cup milk of your choice
- 1/2 cup maple syrup
- 2 tablespoons raw cocoa powder
- 1 teaspoon vanilla extract
- Pinch of salt

Directions

1. Add hazelnuts to a food processor and blend them until they are broken down nicely. The longer you process, the better the final product will be, but I usually don't have enough patience and blend them for 2-3 minutes. You may need to stop a few times and scrape the sides of the processor with a spatula.
2. Add milk, maple syrup, cocoa, vanilla and salt and blend for another one or two minutes, until it gets nice and smooth.
3. Store in an airtight container in the fridge for about 2 weeks.

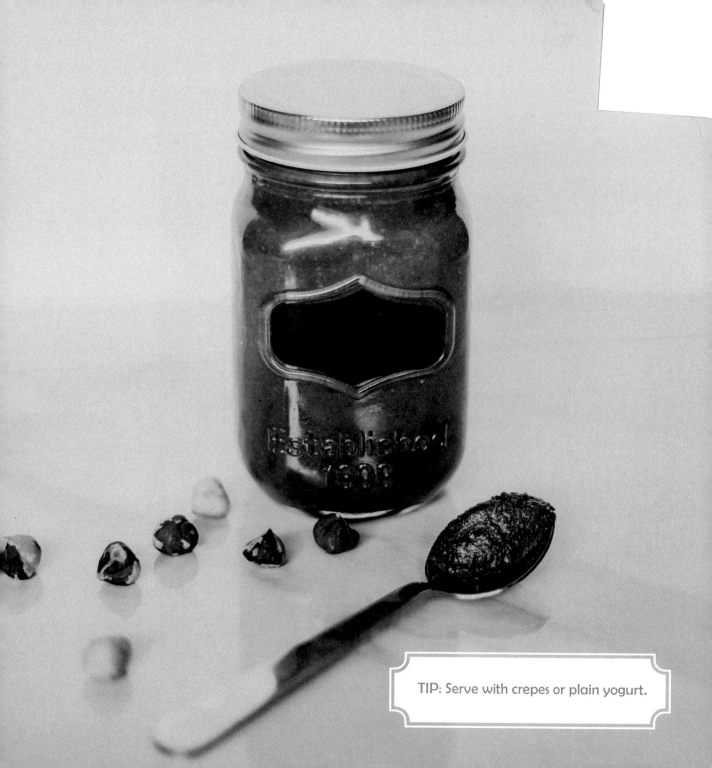

TIP: Serve with crepes or plain yogurt.

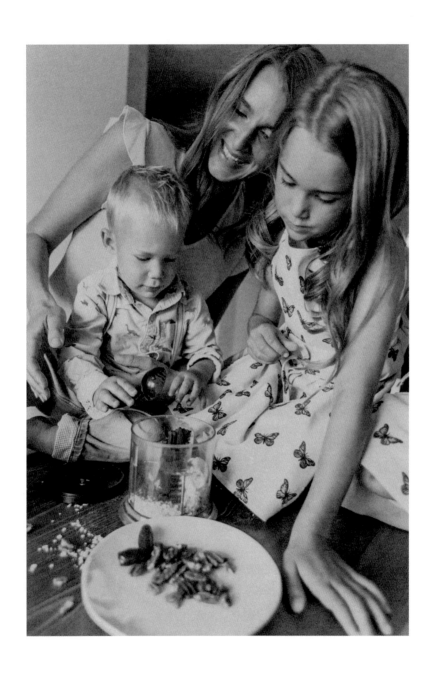

Muffins

Muffins have a bad reputation for being very high in calories, fat and sugar. But not these! The recipes in this section are made with nuts and nut or seed butter without the addition of any flour. They are sweetened by fruit, so they are naturally sugar-free!

Muffins are one of our most favorite things to bake. They are easy to make and my kids love to add toppings on top of each muffin. They are a convenient snack on the go, and easy to take to play dates or pack for a school lunch.

I love using foil-lined baking cups to make sure my muffins don't stick to the tin or to the baking cup, as regular paper cups tend to do. It's easier for kids to remove the cup, plus it saves me time greasing and then cleaning the tin!

All the muffins in this section should be stored in an airtight container at cool room temperature for up to 2 days, in the refrigerator for up to 1 week, or the freezer for up to 3 months.

Healthy Mighty Muffins

Sugar-free, Gluten-free, Dairy-free

This is one of our favorite muffin recipes of all time! I can't take credit for this recipe as it was developed by my friend Lindsay Gee. Lindsay has a PhD in Exercise Physiology and works hard to help others feel healthy and strong through fitness and nutrition. She is a health warrior, mental health advocate, writer and creator of many fitness programs designed to improve both physical and mental health. Check her out!

Ingredients

- 1 cup dates, pitted
- 1 cup almond butter (or nut/seed butter of choice)
- 2 ripe bananas
- 3 eggs
- 1 teaspoon baking soda
- 1 teaspoon cinnamon
- Pinch of salt
- 1/4 cup chia seeds

Add-ins & toppings

1/2 cup sunflower seeds
1/2 cup chopped walnuts, pecans or almonds
1/2 cup any unsweetened dried fruit
1/2 cup berries
1/2 cup chocolate chips

Directions

1. Preheat oven to 350°F/180°C and line a muffin pan with baking cups.
2. In a microwave-safe bowl, cover dates with water. Microwave for 1-1½ minutes to soften the dates. Strain the water.
3. Blend the dates in a food processor until smooth. Add almond butter, bananas, eggs, baking soda, sea salt and cinnamon and blend until fully combined. Stir in chia seeds and any add-ins you choose.
4. Fill each muffin cup with the mixture. Top with topping of your choice, if desired. Bake for 15-20 minutes, until toothpick comes out clean.

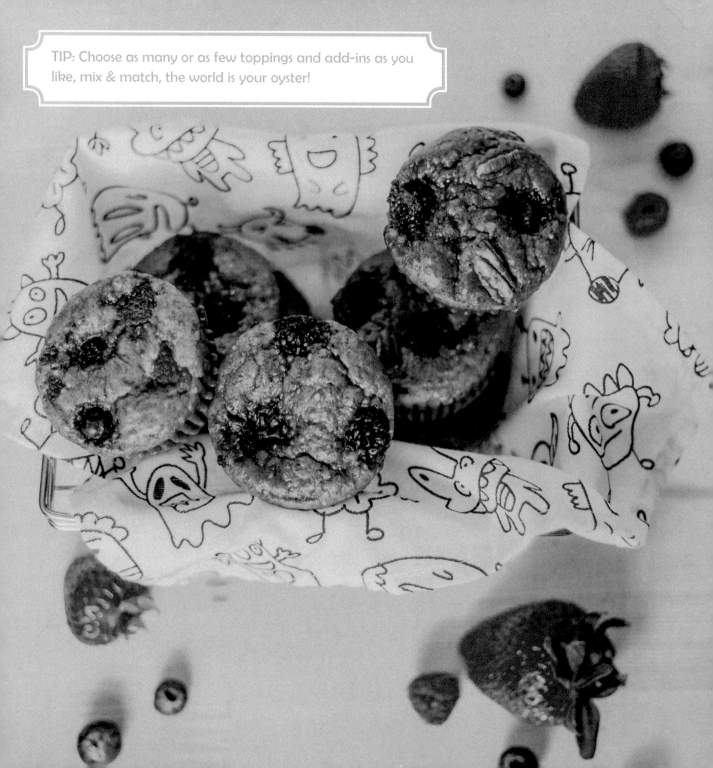

TIP: Choose as many or as few toppings and add-ins as you like, mix & match, the world is your oyster!

Lemon Poppyseed Muffins

Sugar-free, Gluten-free, Dairy-free

These are my personal favorites and my kids and husband approved! Poppyseeds are one of the most commonly used ingredients for baking in Europe. They are high in calcium (helps build strong bones), iron (promotes a healthy immune system) and zinc (promotes healthy skin, hair nails, and has a number of other benefits). But my favorite part is that poppyseeds are proven to help with good mood! And in case you were wondering, the opiate is removed when poppyseeds are processed, so they are perfectly safe for your whole family to eat!

Ingredients

- 1 & 1/2 cup natural cashews (or almonds)
- 1 cup dates, pitted
- 1/2 lemon (juice and zest)
- 3 eggs
- 1 teaspoon vanilla extract
- 1/2 teaspoon baking soda
- Pinch of salt
- 1/4 cup poppy seeds

Directions

1. Preheat oven to 350°F/180°C and line a muffin pan with baking cups.
2. In a food processor, blend cashews until finely ground.
3. In a microwave-safe bowl, cover dates with water and microwave for 1 minute. Strain the water. Add the dates into the food process and blend with cashews until a crumbly texture is formed.
4. Add lemon juice, zest, egg, vanilla extract, baking soda and salt and process until everything is well combined. Stir in poppy seeds.
5. Fill each muffin cup with the mixture. Bake for around 15-20 minutes, until toothpick comes out clean.

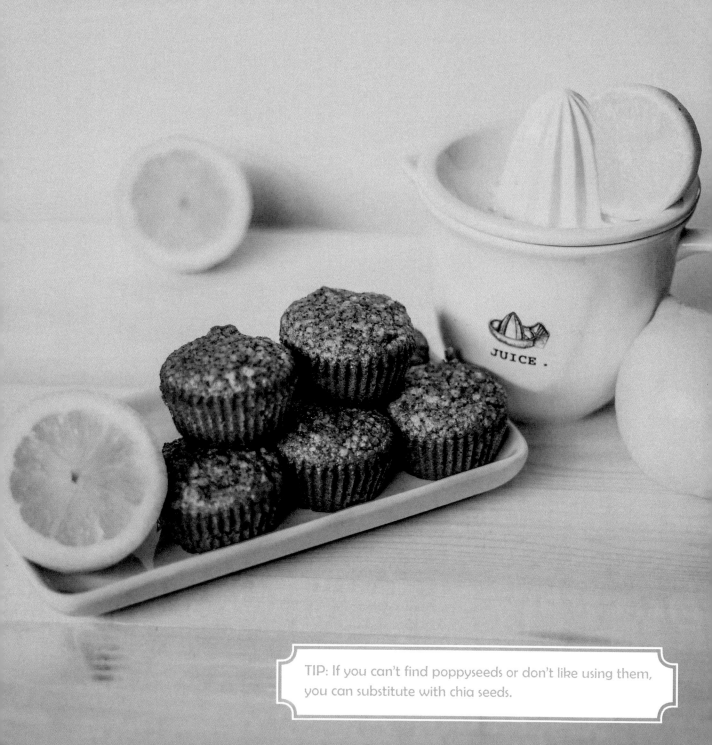

TIP: If you can't find poppyseeds or don't like using them, you can substitute with chia seeds.

Plant-Based Nut-Free Apple Muffins

Sugar-free, Gluten-free, Dairy-free, Vegan, Nut-free

These muffins are a great addition for kids' lunch boxes for a nut-free environment, or a great snack on the go for the whole family! They are plant-based and friendly for most common allergies. Grab one from the freezer before leaving the house and they are thawed and ready to eat for an afternoon snack.

Ingredients

- 1 cup prunes (or pitted dates)
- 1 cup pumpkin seed butter (or seed butter of your choice)
- 2 tablespoons ground flaxseed
- 1/2 cup applesauce, unsweetened
- 2 ripe bananas
- 1 teaspoon baking soda
- 1 teaspoon cinnamon
- 1 cup diced apple

Directions

1. Preheat oven to 350°F/180°C and line a muffin pan with baking cups.
2. Put prunes into a food processor and process until smooth. Add pumpkin butter, flaxseeds, applesauce, bananas, baking soda, cinnamon, ginger, cloves and pinch of salt and blend until everything is well combined. Stir in apple (don't blend).
3. Fill each muffin cup with the mixture. Bake for around 20-25 minutes, until brown around the edges and the muffins feel firmer.

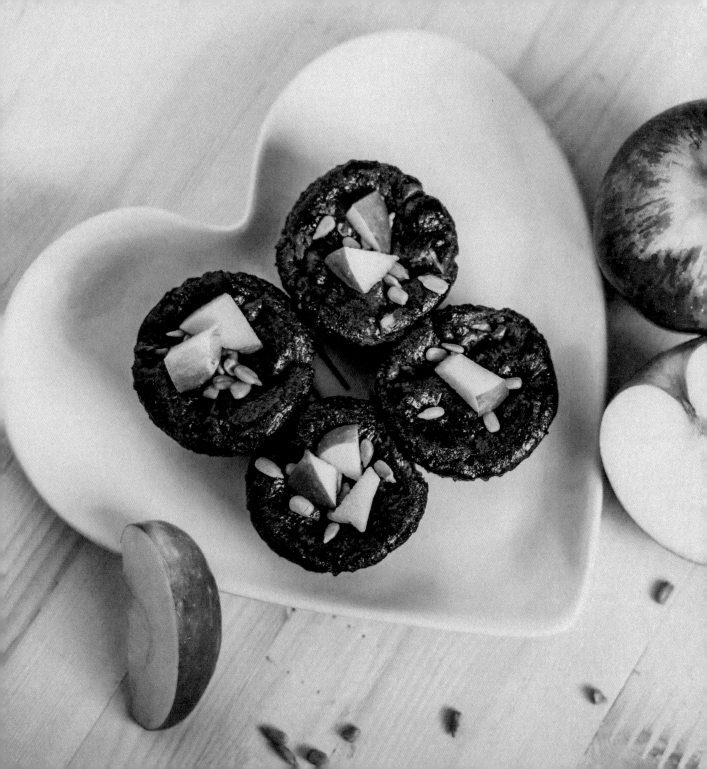

Carrot Cake Muffins

Sugar-free, Gluten-free, Dairy-free

Healthy muffins that taste like carrot cake. Oh, yes please! Turn these into a cupcakes by adding unsweetened homemade whipped cream on top, or serve as a snack for kids with natural plain yogurt.

Ingredients

- 1 cup dates, pitted
- 1/2 cup natural almonds
- 1/2 cup natural walnuts
- 1 cup grated carrots (about 3 medium carrots)
- 3 eggs
- 1/4 cup shredded coconut
- 1/2 teaspoon grated fresh ginger (or 1/4 teaspoon ground ginger)
- 1/2 teaspoon cinnamon
- Pinch of salt

Directions

1. Preheat oven to 350°F/180°C and line a muffin pan with baking cups.
2. In a microwave-safe bowl, cover dates with water. Microwave for 1 minute to soften the dates. Strain the water and set aside.
3. Grate carrots on a grater or in a food processor. If using food processor, don't overprocess. Set aside.
4. Blend almonds and walnuts in a food processor until finely ground. Add softened dates and blend until dates are fully processed. Add eggs and blend until the mixture is smooth.
5. Stir in grated carrots, shredded coconut and spices (ginger, cinnamon and salt). Make sure everything is nicely combined.
6. Fill each muffin cup with the mixture. Bake for around 20 minutes, until toothpick comes out clean.

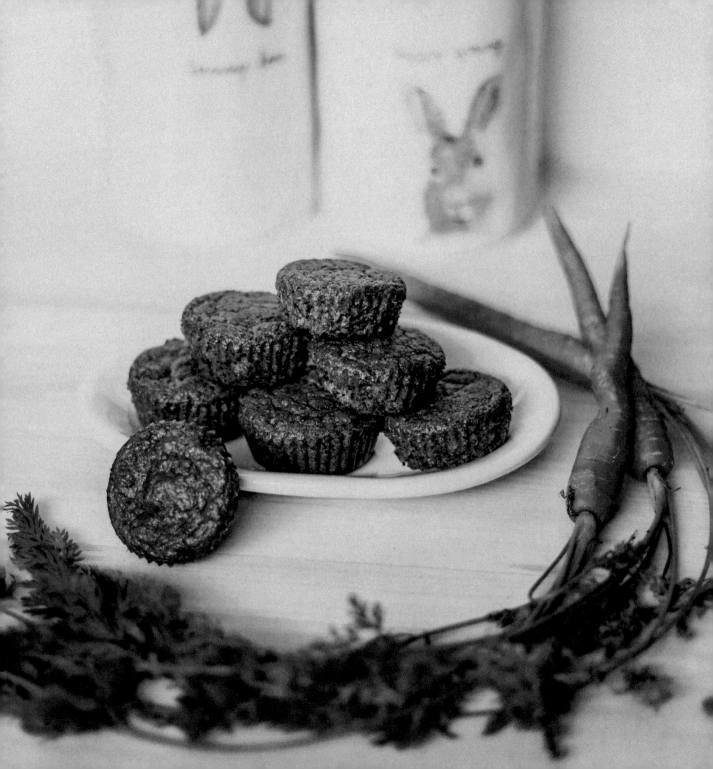

Blueberry Mini Muffins

Sugar-free, Gluten-free, Nut-free

Blueberries are one of my favorite fruit to keep on hand in a freezer. I usually have all of these ingredients in my pantry, so I'm ready to whip up these mini muffins at any time.

Ingredients

- 1/2 cup dates, pitted
- 1/2 cup oats (certified gluten-free, as needed)
- 1/4 cup natural plain yogurt
- 2 eggs
- 1/4 cup blueberries
- 1 teaspoon vanilla extract
- 1/2 teaspoon baking soda
- Pinch of salt
- 24 blueberries to top

Directions

1. Preheat oven to 350°F/180°C and line a 24-mini-muffin tin with mini-muffin baking cups.
2. In a microwave-safe bowl, cover dates with water and microwave for 1 minute. Strain the water and put aside.
3. In a food processor, blend oats until ground. Add softened dates and blend until combined. Add rest of the ingredients—yogurt, eggs, blueberries, vanilla extract, baking soda and salt, and blend until smooth.
4. Fill each mini-muffin cup with the mixture. Top with blueberries. Bake for around 20 minutes, until toothpick comes out clean.

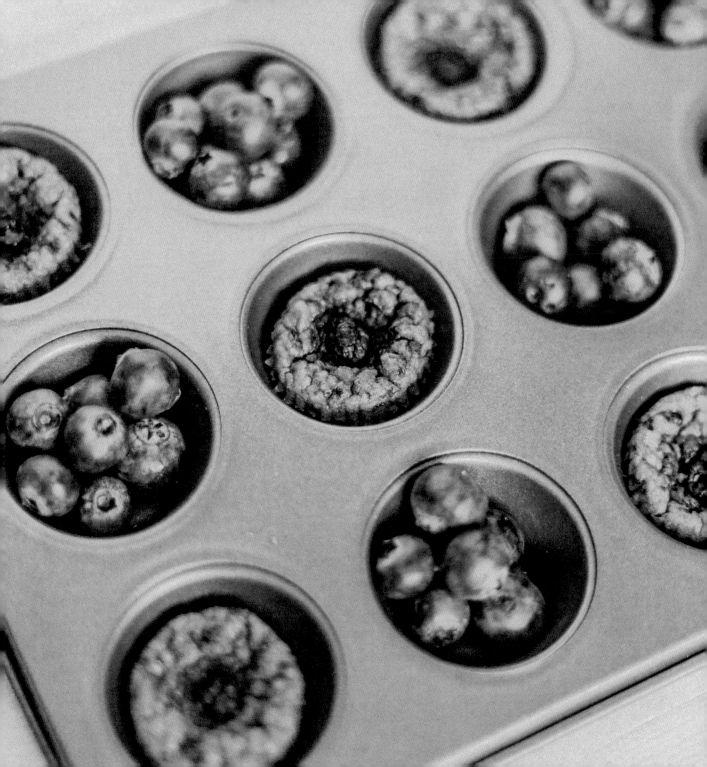

Monkey's Favorite Mini Muffins

Gluten-free, Dairy-free

My oldest daughter, Ariana, has a favorite stuffy she's carried around since her first Christmas—a monkey. Her monkey loves bananas, peanut butter and chocolate chips, so naturally, these mini muffins are her monkey's favorite! They are super simple and my kids love to bake these with me! Their favorite part is to add chocolate chips on top of each muffin (and a few in their mouth).

Ingredients

- 1/2 cup dates, pitted
- 1 ripe banana
- 2 eggs
- 1/2 cup creamy natural peanut butter (or other nut butter of choice)
- 1 tablespoon coconut oil, melted
- 1 teaspoon vanilla extract
- 1/2 teaspoon baking soda
- Pinch of salt
- Handful of mini chocolate chips (optional, dairy-free as needed)

Directions

1. Preheat oven to 350°F/180°C and line a 24-mini-muffin tin with mini-muffin baking cups.
2. In a microwave-safe bowl, cover dates with water and microwave for 1 minute to soften. Strain the water. Add the softened dates, banana, eggs, peanut butter, coconut oil, vanilla, baking soda and salt to your food processor. Process until a smooth puree.
3. Fill each mini-muffin cup with the mixture. Sprinkle chocolate chips on top of each muffin.
4. Bake for around 15 minutes, until toothpick comes out clean.

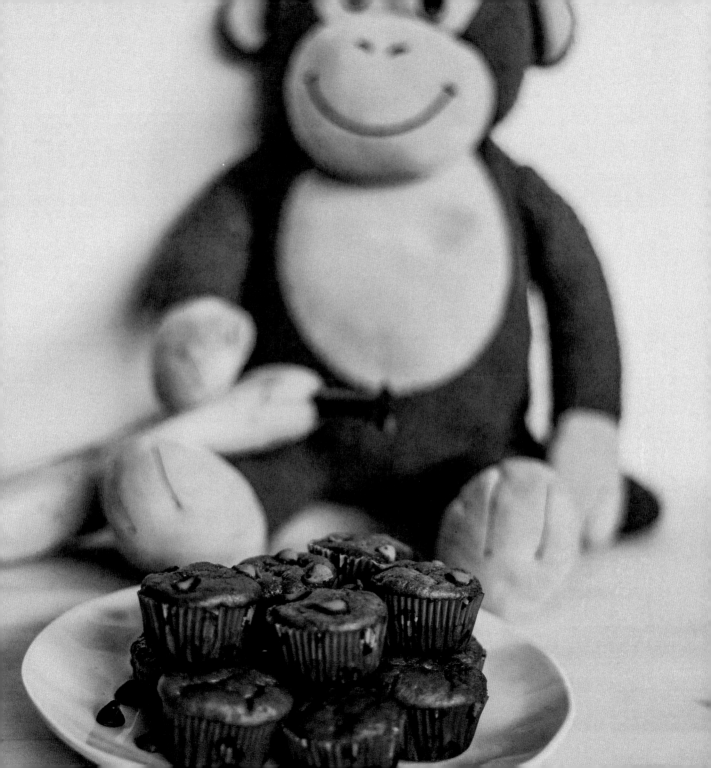

Piña Colada Mini Muffins

Sugar-free, Gluten-free, Dairy-free, Nut-free

The combination of coconut and pineapple always brings back memories of vacationing by a pool with a drink in my hand. Since the winter is way too long, I love to bring this memory back often. I wish I could add rum to these (just kidding . . . or not. Don't judge me!).

Ingredients

- 1/2 cup oats (certified gluten-free, as needed)
- 1 ripe banana
- 1/4 cup coconut cream (see page 15 for how to get the coconut cream)
- 2 eggs
- 1/4 cup shredded coconut, unsweetened
- 1 teaspoon vanilla extract
- 1/2 teaspoon baking soda
- Pinch of salt
- Small pieces of pineapple for topping (about 1/2 cup)

Directions

1. Preheat oven to 350°F/180°C and line a 24-mini-muffin tin with mini-muffin baking cups.
2. Blend oats in a food processor until finely ground (flour-like consistency). Add banana, coconut cream, eggs, baking soda, vanilla and pinch of salt and blend well, until fully combined. Stir in shredded coconut and pineapple pieces.
3. Fill each mini-muffin cup with the mixture.
4. Bake for around 15–20 minutes, until toothpick comes out clean.

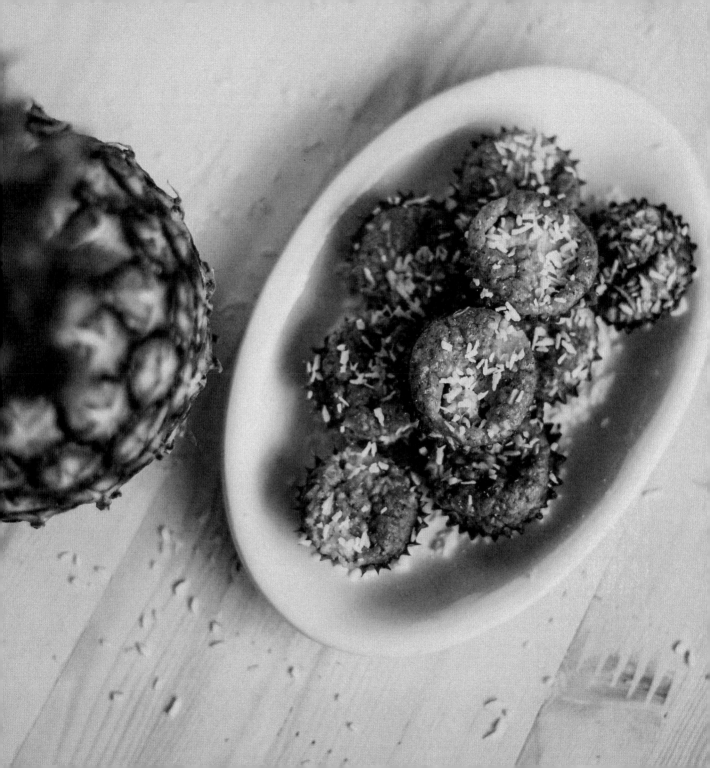

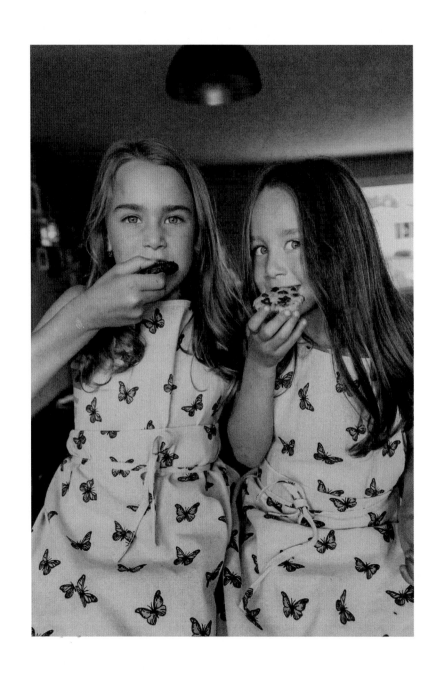

Cookies

As much as kids love cookies, they are not Mom's favorite. No wonder, since they are ranked high on the "junk food" list right next to chips and sweetened drinks. They've earned this spot, since they are commonly made with white bleached flour (zero nutrition), trans fat (for longer shelf life) and a ton of sugar (so they taste good and people will buy them despite the fact that they contain nothing that is good for our bodies).

To this day, my kids actually don't know they can get a free cookie at the grocery store. I'm glad we can make our own cookies that are healthy, flour- oil- and sugar-free. Another mom win right here—turning junk food into nutritional super food!

All cookies in this section should be stored in an airtight container and refrigerated for up to 5 days, or frozen for up to 3 months.

Baby's First Cookie

Sugar-free, Gluten-free, Dairy-free, Vegan, Nut-free

The base for these cookies contains only 2 ingredients and they are perfect for babies who just started to eat solid food. My kids loved to help me make these when they were toddlers! The cookies are so easy to make and they loved to customize their own cookie by adding favorite toppings and flavors.

Ingredients

- 2 ripe bananas (The riper your bananas, the sweeter your cookie will be)
- 1 1/2 cup oats (certified gluten-free, as needed; you can use rolled oats, quick oats or oat flour for a different cookie texture)

Directions

1. Preheat the oven to 350°F/180°C and line a baking tray with parchment paper or a silicone baking sheet.
2. In a large mixing bowl, mash the bananas with fork until smooth. Add the oats and mix until fully combined. Add in any flavors and toppings, if desired.
3. Use your hands to form balls and place onto the baking tray. Flatten a bit with a palm of your hand or fork to create a round cookie shape.
4. Bake for approximately 12 - 15 minutes, or until golden and firmer.

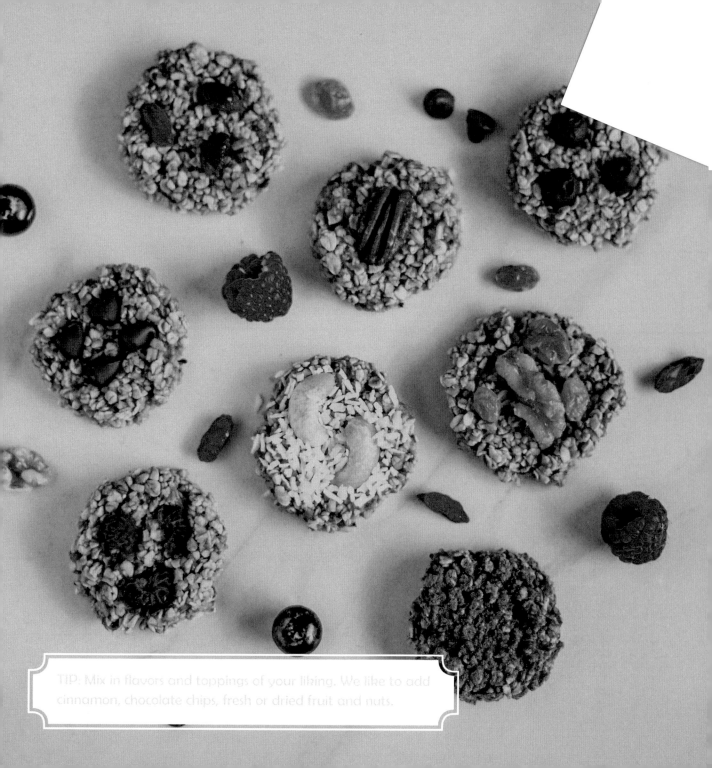

TIP: Mix in flavors and toppings of your liking. We like to add cinnamon, chocolate chips, fresh or dried fruit and nuts.

Delicious Chocolate Walnut Cookies

Sugar-free, Gluten-free, Dairy-free, Vegan

A must-try recipe! Simple, fast and delicious —what else can a busy mom ask for (other than 8 hours of uninterrupted sleep and drinking a coffee while it's still hot, but let's not dream that big)!

Ingredients

- 1 & 1/2 cup walnuts
- 1 cup dates, pitted
- 1 tablespoon raw cocoa powder
- 1/2 teaspoon baking soda
- 1 teaspoon vanilla extract

- 1 teaspoon apple cider vinegar
- Pinch of salt
- 1/2 cup dairy-free chocolate chunks (or chocolate chips of your choice, optional)

Directions

1. Preheat the oven to 350°F/180°C and line a baking sheet with parchment paper or silicone baking mat.
2. In a microwave-safe bowl, cover dates with water and microwave for 1 minute to soften. Keep the water aside.
3. In a food processor, blend walnuts until finely ground. Add the softened dates into the food process and blend with walnuts until a crumbly texture is formed. Add in baking soda, vanilla, salt and vinegar, and process again until the mixture is relatively smooth. If it looks too firm, add little bit of water from the dates. The batter should still be sticky and not runny.
4. Spoon the batter onto a baking sheet and use fork to gently flatten the cookies. I recommend watering the spoon every time to prevent stickiness.
5. Top with chocolate chunks, if desired. Bake for about 15 minutes, until the edges of the cookies start to feel dry. They will still be soft and tender in the middle. Allow to cool for at least 10 minutes before serving.

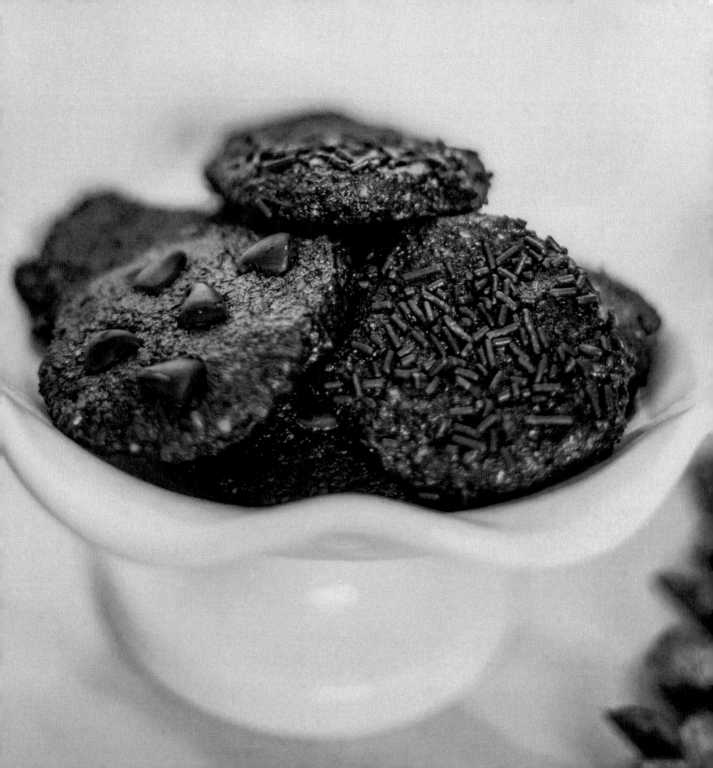

Birthday Cookies

Gluten-free, Dairy-free, Vegan

Yes, I know the sprinkles are sugar. But kids eat with their eyes and the amount of sprinkles is small, considering all the other healthy ingredients. You can omit the sprinkles and replace them with sliced almonds to make almond cookies, if you like.

Ingredients

- 1 cup raw almonds (or nut of your choice)
- 1 cup dates, pitted
- 1/2 cup almond butter (or seed/nut butter of your choice)
- 1 teaspoons vanilla extract
- 1 tablespoon rainbow sprinkles

Directions

1. Preheat the oven to 350°F/180°C and line a baking sheet with parchment paper or silicone baking mat.
2. In a food processor, blend almonds until finely ground. In a microwave-safe bowl, cover dates with water and microwave for 1 minute. Strain the water. Add softened dates into the food processor and blend with almonds. Add almond butter and vanilla extract and blend until everything combined.
3. Spoon the dough onto a baking sheet and use fork to gently flatten the cookies. Top with sprinkles.
4. Bake for 10 minutes, until the edges of the cookies start to feel dry. Allow to cool for at least 10 minutes before serving.

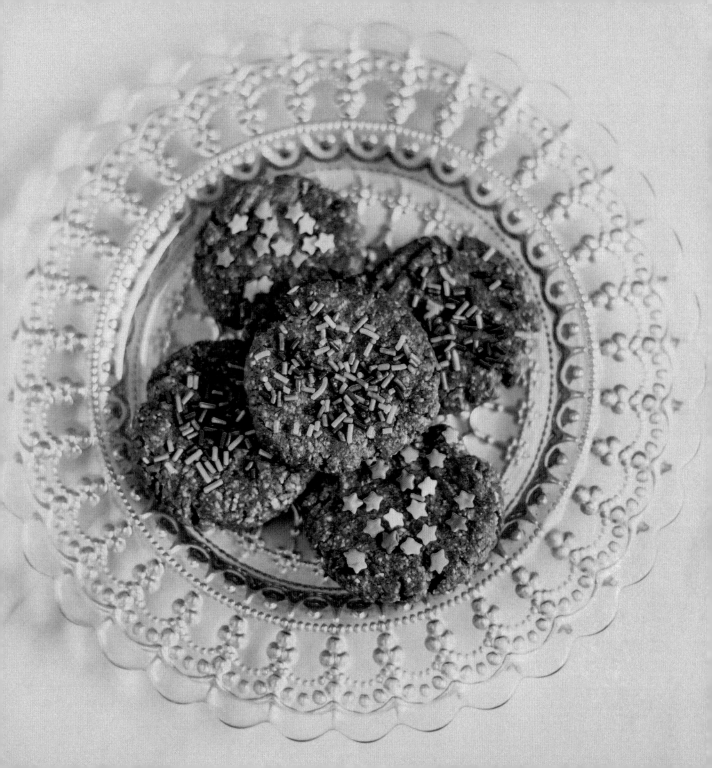

Chocolate-Chip Cookies

Gluten-free, Dairy-free, Nut-free

How could I create a cookie section in my cookbook and not include a chocolate-chip cookie recipe? My husband loves chocolate-chip cookies. I should tell you, he loves his cookie to be loaded with chocolate and more chocolate, so I tried to create a recipe that would satisfy his cravings. Now, this may not be the healthiest recipe in my book, but it is still a much healthier version than regular chocolate-chip cookies. Everything in moderation, right? Enjoy!

Ingredients

- 1 & 1/2 cup oats (certified gluten-free, as needed)
- 1/4 cup coconut oil, melted
- 1 egg
- 1 tablespoon maple syrup
- 2 teaspoons vanilla extract
- Pinch of salt
- 1/2 cup dairy-free chocolate chunks (or chocolate chips of your choice)

Directions

1. Preheat oven to 350°F/180°C and line a baking tray with parchment paper or silicone baking sheet.
2. Blend oats in a food processor until finely ground (flour-like consistency). Add melted coconut oil, egg, vanilla extract, maple syrup, baking soda and salt and blend well, until fully combined. Stir in the chocolate chunks.
3. Use your hands to form tight balls or use a cookie scoop and pack tightly, as they may crumble. Place the dough balls onto a parchment sheet and flatten with your palm or spatula.
4. Bake for 10-15 minutes or until lightly browned around the edges. Remove and allow to stay on the baking sheet for at least 10 minutes to cool down. If the cookies are too crumbly, refrigerate them before serving.

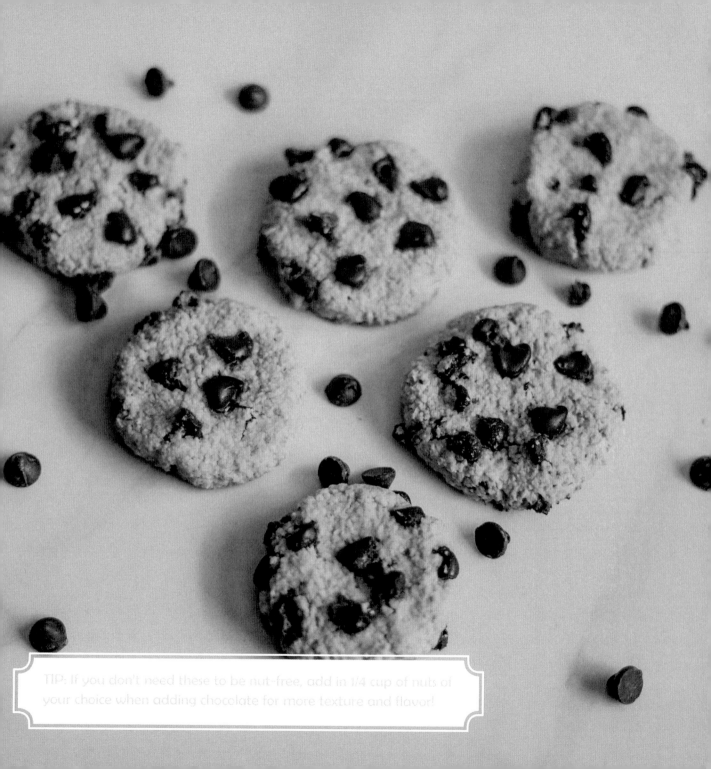

TIP: If you don't need these to be nut-free, add in 1/4 cup of nuts of your choice when adding chocolate for more texture and flavor!

Peanut Butter & Jam Cookies

Gluten-free, Dairy-free

These cookies are so fun to make. My kids love to make the thumbprint in each cookie and then add the jam on top. Plus you can never go wrong with the PB&J combination!

Ingredients

- 1/2 cup oats (certified gluten-free, as needed)
- 1 cup peanut butter
- 1 banana
- 1 egg
- 1 tablespoon maple syrup
- 1 teaspoon vanilla extract
- Pinch of salt
- Berry Chia Jam (recipe on page 36)

Directions

1. Preheat the oven to 350°F/180°C and line a baking tray with parchment paper or silicone baking sheet.
2. Blend oats in a food processor until finely ground (flour-like consistency). Add in the peanut butter, banana, egg, maple syrup, vanilla and salt. Process until a sticky, uniform batter is created. Scrape down the food processor to ensure that everything gets thoroughly mixed.
3. Use your hands to form a ball. If the batter is too sticky, wet your hands before rolling each ball. Place balls onto the baking sheet. Gently press the balls with your (or a child's) thumb to make a small well-like indent. It helps to wet the thumb each time you press the cookie.
4. Add a spoonful of Berry Chia Jam to the thumbprint.
5. Bake for 15-20 minutes, until the edges of the cookies start to feel dry. Allow the cookies to cool completely before removing them from the baking sheet.

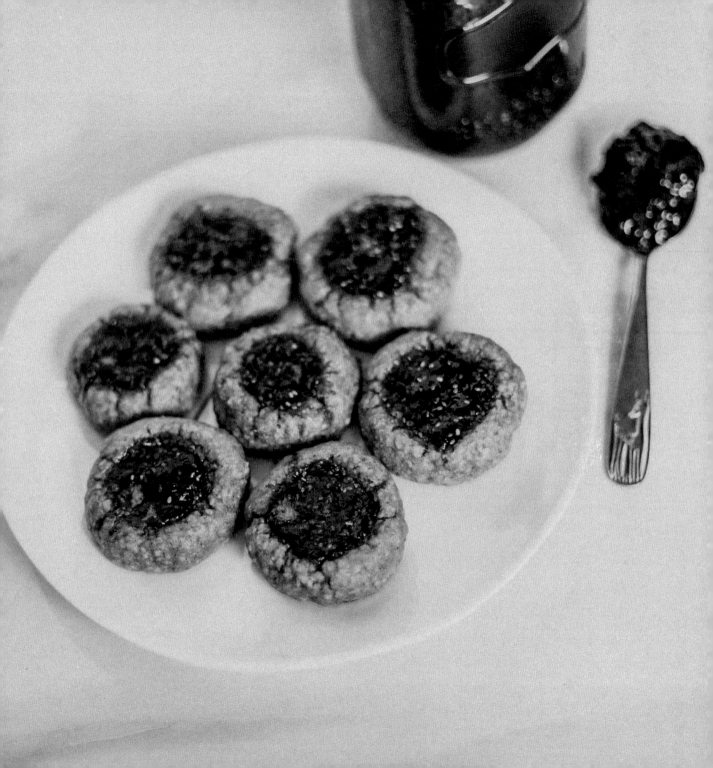

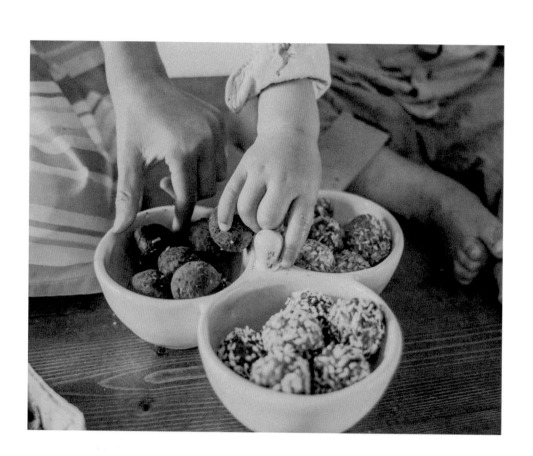

Bliss Balls

What are bliss balls, you ask? Only the most convenient, easiest, fastest and most nutrition-packed snack ever invented! Bliss balls are basically a blend of dried fruit, seeds and nuts rolled into a ball shape and then coated in coconut or nuts. They are very easy to make, no baking required, and are a great snack on the go!

The fruit, nut and seed combination found in these balls means that they are jam-packed with fiber. This fiber is going to help keep your blood sugar levels stable and will help fill you up so you are not ravenously hungry 20 minutes after eating.

These nutritional heroes include good fats, natural protein and healthy carbs, and are free of additives, preservatives, and common allergens like wheat, gluten, dairy, soy, eggs, etc. I also included a few nut-free options. If you are doing meal prep, these are so handy to make and you will have them for the rest of the week. They make a great post-workout snack for you, or an after-gym snack for your kiddos to refuel their energy and keep them going for the rest of the day!

All these recipes make around 15-20 balls, which should be stored in the fridge in an airtight container for up to a week, or frozen for up to 3 months.

Energy Bliss Balls

Sugar-free, Gluten-free, Dairy-free, Vegan, Raw

These bliss balls will definitely hit your sweet spot! Containing nutrient-dense chia seeds and hempseeds, they are the perfect snack after any physical activity.

Ingredients

- 1/2 cup dates, pitted
- 1/2 cup almonds
- 1/2 cup hazelnuts
- 1 tablespoon chia seeds

- 1 tablespoon raw cocoa powder
- 1 teaspoon vanilla extract
- Pinch of salt
- Hempseeds for coating

Directions

1. In a microwave-safe bowl, cover dates with water. Microwave for 1 minute to soften the dates.
2. In a food processor, blend almonds and hazelnuts until finely ground.
3. Add remaining ingredients—softened dates, chia seeds, cocoa powder, vanilla extract and salt. Blend well until everything is combined. You may need to scrape the food processor with a spatula a few times and blend again.
4. Using wet hands, roll tablespoons of the mixture into snack-sized balls and roll in the hempseeds to coat.
5. Place the balls on the tray or plate and refrigerate for 30 minutes before serving.

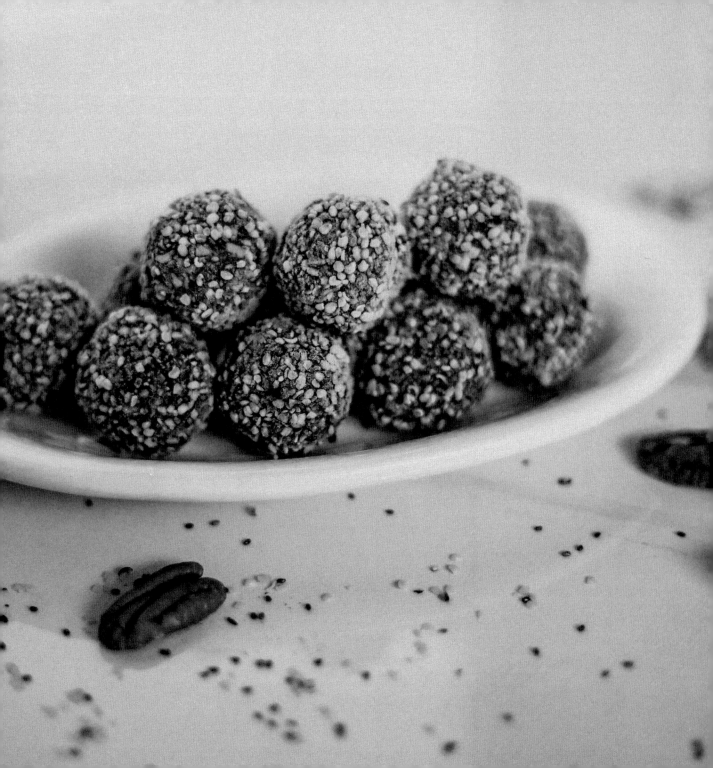

Lemon Poppy Seed Bliss Balls

Sugar-free, Gluten-free, Dairy-free, Vegan, Raw

If you tried my lemon poppy seed muffins, you know how much I love this combination. But I don't love baking in the summer on hot days (hence, all the bliss ball and raw cake recipes). I wanted to recreate the muffins without turning the oven on. These are equally good and became one of our favorite bliss balls.

Ingredients

- 1 cup cashews (or almonds)
- 1/2 cup golden raisins
- 1/4 cup poppy seeds
- 1/2 lemon (juice and zest)
- 1 tablespoon coconut oil, melted
- 1 tablespoon vanilla extract
- Pinch of salt

Directions

1. In a food processor, blend cashews until finely ground. Add raisins and blend until combined.
2. Add remaining ingredients—poppy seeds, lemon juice and zest, melted coconut oil, vanilla extract and salt. Blend until combined and crumbly consistency is created.
3. Roll into balls and enjoy immediately or refrigerate before serving.

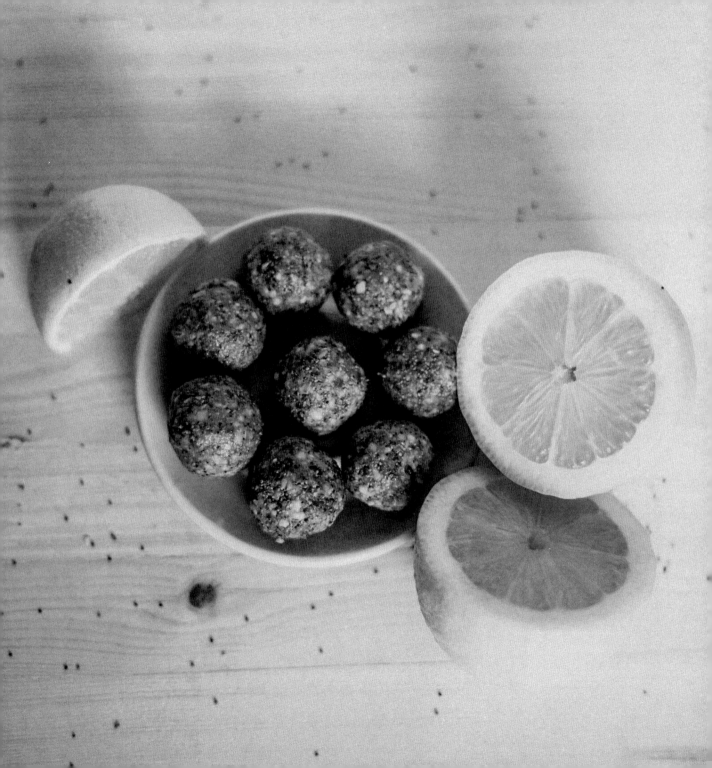

Strawberry Cheesecake Bliss Balls

Sugar-free, Gluten-free, Nut-free, Raw

With most schools having a strict nut-free policy, I was trying to create a nut-free version of bliss balls. I recommend storing them in a freezer, popping them into your child's lunch box in the morning, and they will melt just in time for a lunch treat! These are also perfect for a hot summer day, slowly melting in your mouth as you eat them. Make sure to use frozen strawberries, otherwise the mixture will be too runny and you won't be able to roll them into balls. If that happens, turn them into popsicles by pouring the mixture into popsicle molds and freezing until firm!

Ingredients

- 1 cup strawberries, frozen
- 1/2 cup cream cheese (or dry cottage cheese)
- 1/2 cup shredded coconut, unsweetened
- 1 teaspoon lemon juice
- 1 teaspoon vanilla extract
- Extra shredded coconut for coating

Directions

1. In a food processor, blend all ingredients—frozen strawberries, cream cheese, shredded coconut, lemon juice and vanilla extract.
2. Blend until the strawberries are chopped and throughout the cheese cream. It should be thick, not runny, partially frozen. Don't overprocess.
3. Roll into balls and coat in coconut.

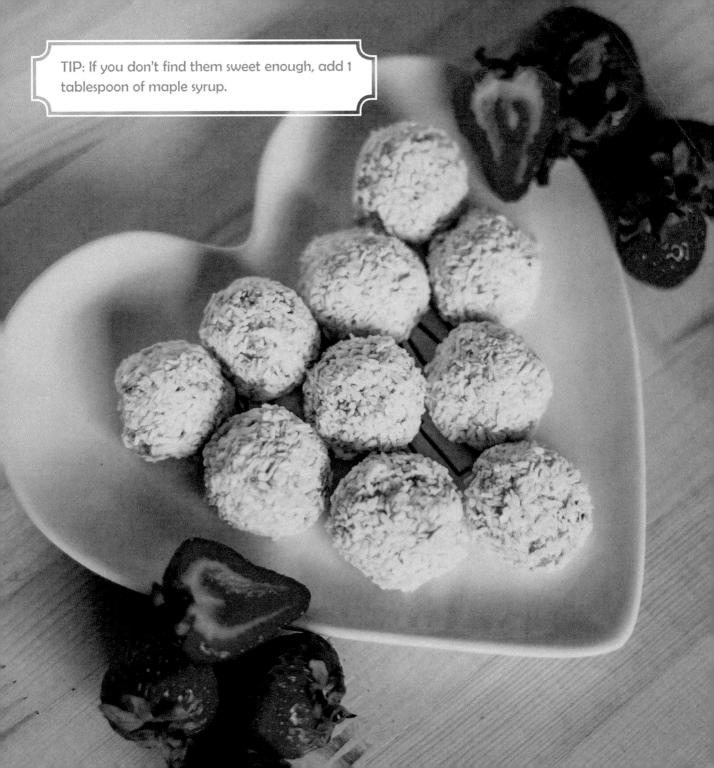

TIP: If you don't find them sweet enough, add 1 tablespoon of maple syrup.

Chocolate Mint Bliss Balls

Sugar-free, Gluten-free, Dairy-free, Vegan, Raw

You can make these with any nuts of your liking, or any nuts that you currently have in your pantry. It is recommended to alternate nuts you eat, since every nut has different nutritional value and vitamins.

Ingredients

- 1 & 1/2 cup nuts (any of these: cashews, hazelnuts, macadamia nuts, almonds, pecans or walnuts)
- 1/2 cup dates, pitted
- 1 tablespoon raw cocoa powder
- 1 tablespoon mint extract
- Raw cocoa powder for coating

Directions

1. In a microwave-safe bowl, cover dates with water. Microwave for 1 minute to soften the dates. Set aside.
2. In a food processor, blend nuts of your choice until they break down into crumbs. Add the softened dates, cocoa powder and mint extract. Blend until fully combined.
3. Roll into small balls and coat in raw cocoa powder. Place the balls on the tray or plate and refrigerate for at least 30 minutes.

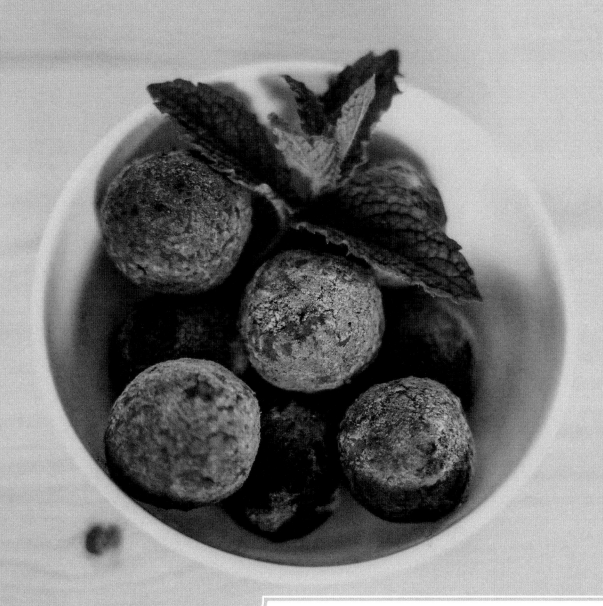

TIP: You can stir in mini chocolate chips for extra chocolatiness (is that even a word? If not, it should be!).

Carrot Cake Bliss Balls

Sugar-free, Gluten-free, Dairy-free, Vegan, Raw

All the taste of carrot cake turned into a bliss ball! I highly recommend using fresh ginger in this recipe for the taste to come out.

Ingredients

- 1/2 cup dates, pitted
- 1/4 cup natural almonds
- 1/4 cup natural walnuts
- 1/2 cup grated carrots (2-3 medium carrots)
- 1/4 cup shredded coconut
- 1/2 teaspoon grated fresh ginger (or 1/4 teaspoon ground ginger)
- 1/2 teaspoon cinnamon
- Pinch of salt
- Extra shredded coconut for coating

Instructions

1. In a microwave-safe bowl, cover dates with water. Microwave for 1 minute to soften the dates and set aside.
2. Grate carrots on a grater or in a food processor. If using food processor, don't overprocess, as you want to keep some texture and not create a puree. Set aside.
3. In a food processor, blend almonds and walnuts until finely ground. Add softened dates and blend until dates are fully processed. Stir in grated carrots, shredded coconut, ginger, cinnamon and salt.
4. Roll into small balls. The mixture may look too dry, but when you start pressing it together in your hands, it will stick together. If the mixture is still too dry and doesn't stick, add a tablespoon of water from dates and pulse one more time. Coat with shredded coconut.

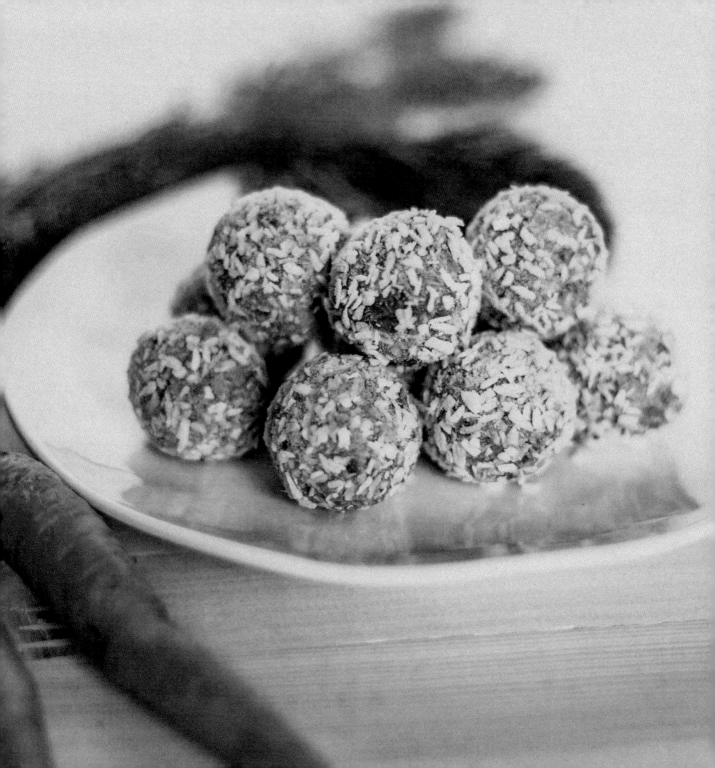

Nut-Free Chocolate Bliss Balls

Sugar-free, Gluten-free, Dairy-free, Vegan, Nut-free, Raw

If you are looking for a perfect snack to bring to a kids' party, look no further! The combination of dates and raisins makes these balls very sweet (they are actually too sweet for me), but very popular with children. And they are gluten-free, dairy-free, nut-free AND sugar-free (Supermom win!).

Ingredients

- 1 cup dates, pitted
- 1 cup sunflower seeds
- 1/2 cup raisins
- 1 tablespoon raw cocoa powder
- 1 tablespoon coconut oil
- Extra shredded coconut for coating

Directions

1. In a microwave-safe bowl, cover dates with water. Microwave for 1 minute to soften the dates. Strain the water.
2. In a food processor, blend sunflower seeds, softened dates, raisins, cocoa powder and melted coconut oil. Blend well, until everything is combined. You may need to scrape the food processor with spatula a few times and blend again.
3. Roll into small balls and coat with shredded coconut. Place the balls on a tray or plate and refrigerate for at least 30 minutes.

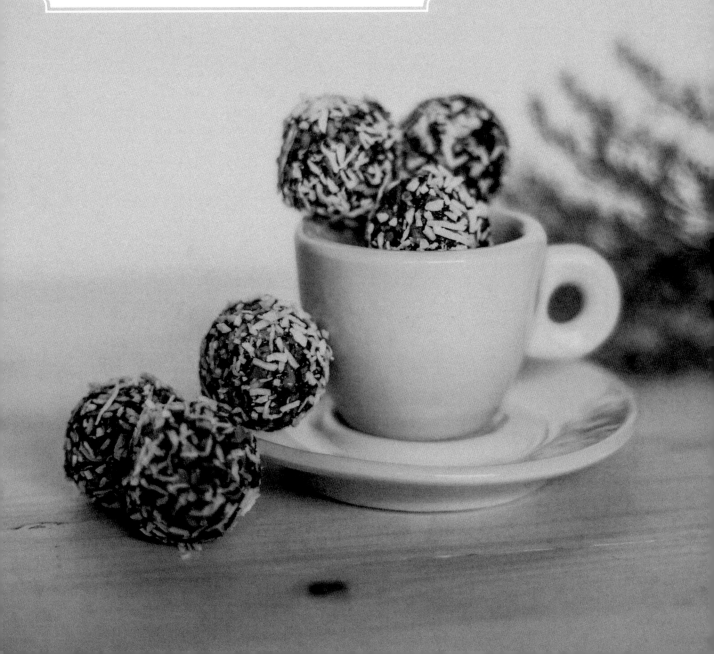

TIP: Add 1/2 cup of mini chocolate chips before rolling into balls to make them extra pleasing. Event kids who are not used to "healthy" eating won't say no to these!

Cherry Bliss Balls

Sugar-free, Gluten-free, Dairy-free, Vegan, Raw

These bliss balls are actually a modified recipe from our traditional Christmas recipe. We would make an adult version by adding rum. (No, I didn't make that up . . . I wasn't joking when I mentioned adding rum to baking. It's a tradition in our small eastern European country!)

Ingredients

- 1/2 cup dates, pitted
- 1 cup walnuts (or 1/2 cup walnuts and 1/2 cup pecans)
- 1 cup frozen cherries, pitted
- 1/2 cup shredded coconut, unsweetened
- 2 tablespoons raw cocoa powder
- Crushed walnuts or pecans for coating

Directions

1. In a microwave-safe bowl, cover dates with water. Microwave for 1 minute to soften the dates. Strain water and set aside.
2. In a food processor, blend walnuts until finely ground. Add softened dates, frozen cherries and cocoa powder and blend until everything is finely chopped and the mixture comes together. Stir in shredded coconut.
3. Roll into small balls and coat with crushed nuts. Place the balls on a tray or plate and refrigerate for at least 30 minutes.

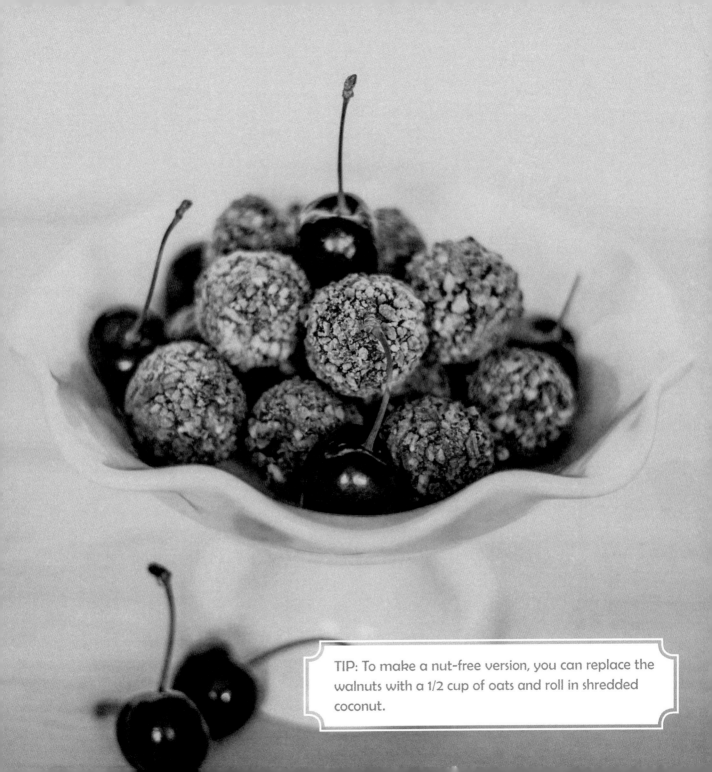

TIP: To make a nut-free version, you can replace the walnuts with a 1/2 cup of oats and roll in shredded coconut.

Simple 3-Ingredient Blueberry Balls

Sugar-free, Gluten-free, Dairy-free, Vegan, Raw

Blueberries are one of our favorite fruit. As mentioned at the beginning of this book, I prefer buying seasonal fruit and eating it fresh, but I always stock up on organic frozen fruit. It is usually cheaper than fresh and has many other benefits, so these bliss balls can be whipped up from ingredients we always have on hand in a few minutes.

Ingredients

- 1 cup oats (certified gluten-free, as needed)
- 1 cup frozen blueberries
- 2 tablespoons peanut butter (or nut butter of choice)

Directions

1. Put oats, blueberries and peanut butter into a food processor and blend until you have a thick mixture (partially still frozen).
2. Form into balls.
3. Store in fridge in an airtight container for up to a week or freeze for up to 3 months.

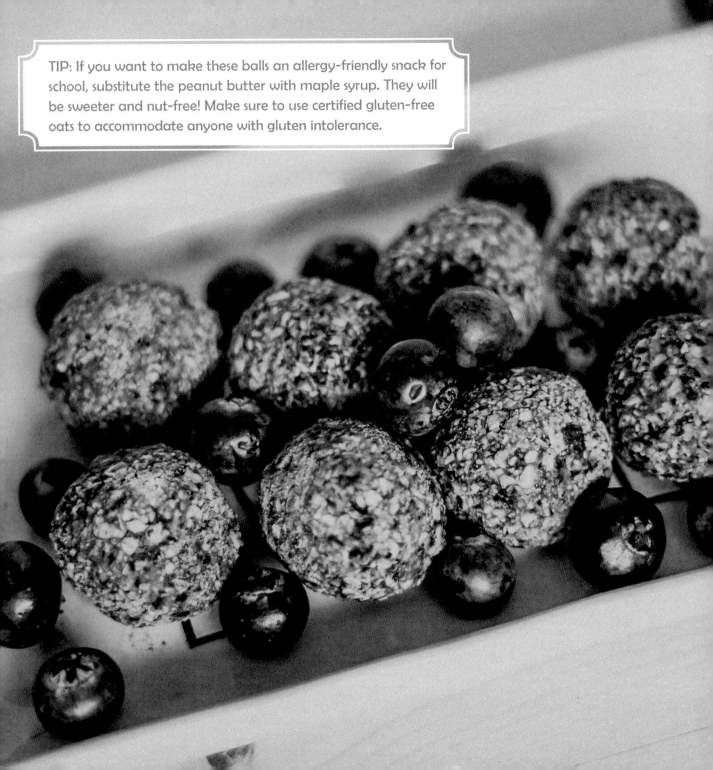

TIP: If you want to make these balls an allergy-friendly snack for school, substitute the peanut butter with maple syrup. They will be sweeter and nut-free! Make sure to use certified gluten-free oats to accommodate anyone with gluten intolerance.

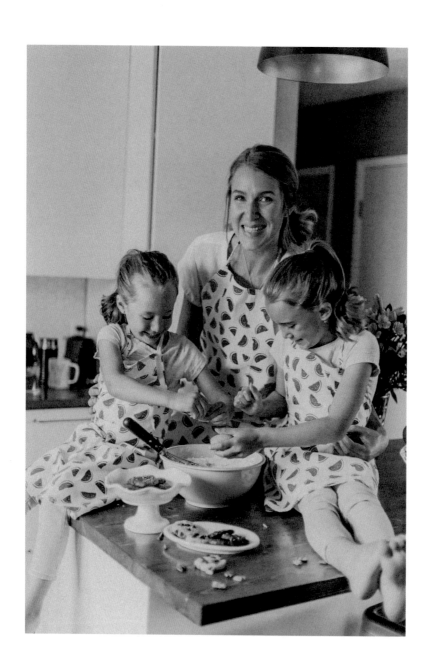

Cakes & More

In this section you will find our favorite cakes and cheesecakes. These are not your traditional cakes, as they are raw and plant-based. These vegan raw cakes changed my perspective on how I look at baked goods and treats in general. They are truly a treat you can feel good about, light in consistency, and you can taste the actual ingredients with their natural sweetness.

Here you will find my favorite peanut butter cups, my husband's favorite banana bread and a few other recipes that are (as always) easy to make using whole food natural ingredients.

The very first recipe in this section is everyone's all-time favorite and I really encourage you to try it!

Love Berry Cheesecake

Sugar-free, Gluten-free, Dairy-free, Vegan, Raw

This is my all-time favorite recipe! Everyone who ever tried it, loves it. If you make only one recipe from my cookbook, please try this one! When I told my friends I was writing a sugar-free cookbook, their first reaction was "You have to include your berry cheesecake!" So, here it is. The burst of flavors from goji berries, strawberries and raspberries is just amazing! And as a bonus, it is PINK! How can it get any better?

Ingredients

Crust
- 1 cup pecans
- 1 cup walnuts
- 1 cup goji berries (or dates)

Cheesecake layer
- 2 cups natural cashews
- 1/2 cup coconut oil, melted
- 1 & 1/2 cup strawberries
- Juice from 1 lemon
- 1 teaspoon vanilla extract
- 1 & 1/2 cup whole raspberries

Directions

1. Prepare 8" round cake pan with parchment paper on the bottom.
2. Soak the cashews in water for 1 hour. Or for faster approach, cover cashews with water in a microwave-safe bowl and microwave for 5 minutes.
3. To make crust: In a food processor, pulse all the nuts until finely ground. Soften goji berries (or dates) by microwaving covered in water for 1 minute. Strain the water and add the gojis to the food processor. Continue mixing gojis and nuts until crumbs form. Place the mixture to bottom of the round cheesecake pan, pressing firmly and evenly.
4. To make the cheesecake layer: Rinse and strain the cashews and place them into the food processor. Pulse until fine crumbs form. Add melted coconut oil, strawberries and lemon juice and continue processing until a very smooth mixture forms.
5. Put the raspberries on top of the crust and pour over the cashew cheesecake layer to cover.
6. Chill in the fridge overnight or place in freezer to set for at least 2-3 hours. Remove from freezer at least 1 hour before serving. Store covered in fridge for up to 4 days or freeze for up to 3 months.

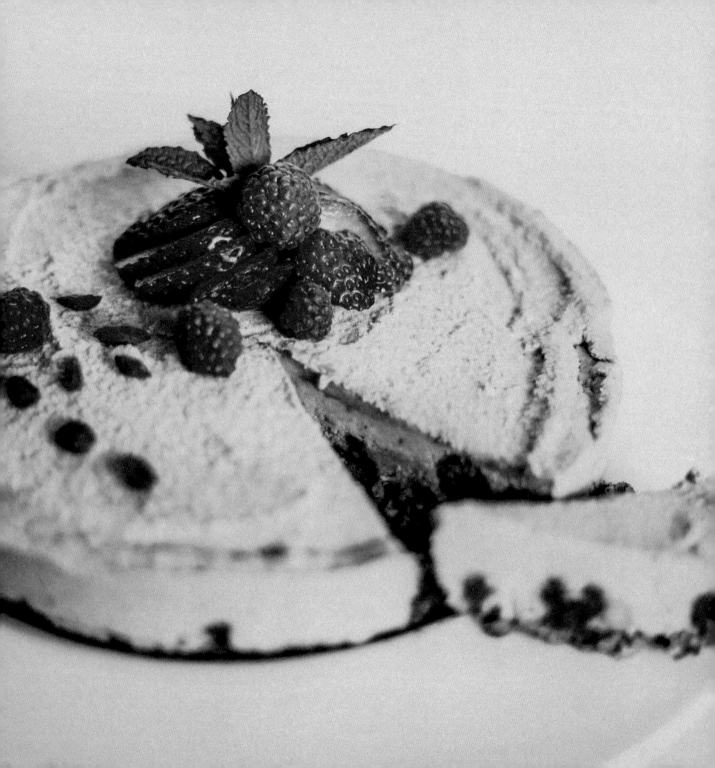

Apple Walnut Cheesecake

Sugar-free, Gluten-free, Dairy-free, Vegan, Raw

This was the very first sugar-free dessert I made, modified from the original recipe a few years ago. After eating this cheesecake, I realized I don't need sugar or sugar substitutes to indulge in a treat. Without the overwhelming sweet taste, you can actually taste all the other ingredients—apples, cinnamon, walnuts and coconut! All the goodness and wholesomeness of simple natural ingredients.

Ingredients

Crust
- 2 bigger apples, grated
- 1 & 1/2 cup walnuts
- 1 cup raisins
- 1/2 cup shredded coconut, unsweetened
- 2 teaspoons cinnamon

Cheesecake layer
- 1 & 1/2 cup natural cashews
- 2 teaspoons lemon juice
- Water, as needed
- Walnuts for decoration

Directions

1. Prepare 8" round cake pan with parchment paper on the bottom.
2. Soak the cashews in water for 1 hour. Or for a faster approach, cover cashews with water in a microwave-safe bowl and microwave for 5 minutes.
3. Wash apples, remove the core and cut them into pieces (leave the skin on).
4. To make crust: In a food processor, pulse all walnuts until finely ground. Add in raisins, apple pieces, coconut and cinnamon and continue blending until crumbs form. Don't overprocess as you want to keep some texture. Spread mixture over bottom of round cheesecake pan, pressing firmly and evenly.
5. To make cheesecake layer: Rinse and strain the cashews and place them into the food processor. Add lemon juice and process on high until a very smooth mixture forms. Add water as needed to create a creamy mixture (about 1-2 tablespoons)
6. Pour the cheesecake layer over the crust. Decorate with walnuts and cinnamon.
7. Chill in the fridge overnight or place in freezer to set for at least 2-3 hours. Remove from freezer 30 minutes before serving. Store covered in fridge for up to 4 days or freeze for up to 3 months.

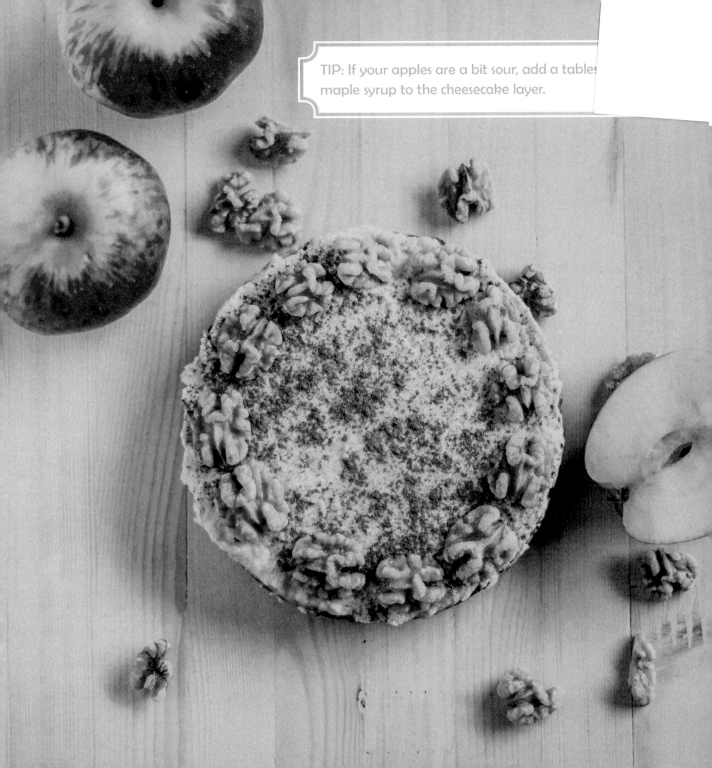

TIP: If your apples are a bit sour, add a tables
maple syrup to the cheesecake layer.

Tropical Sunshine Cake

Sugar-free, Gluten-free, Dairy-free, Vegan, Raw

This sunshine cake is made with mango, coconut and pineapple. The explosion of these flavors brings you right onto a tropical island . . . and it is so sweet, no one will ever guess it contains no sugar whatsoever! Yes, you can have your cake and eat it, too!

Ingredients

Crust

- 3/4 cup dates, pitted
- 1 cup walnuts
- 1/2 cup almonds
- 1/2 cup shredded coconut
- 2 tablespoons raw cocoa powder

Filling

- 1 cup mango (fresh or frozen)
- 1 cup pineapple (fresh or frozen)
- Coconut cream from one can, approx. 1 cup (see page 15 for how to get the coconut cream)
- 1/2 teaspoon vanilla extract
- 1 teaspoon lemon juice
- Handful of shredded coconut to garnish, optional

Directions

1. Prepare 8″ round cake pan with parchment paper on the bottom.
2. In a microwave-safe bowl, cover dates with water and microwave for 1 minute to soften. Set aside.
3. To make crust: In a food processor, pulse walnuts and almonds until finely ground. Add in softened dates and process until combined. Stir in cocoa powder and shredded coconut. Spread mixture over bottom of round pan, pressing firmly and evenly. I use my hands, as the batter is really sticky.
4. To make filling: In a food processor, blend mango, pineapple, coconut cream and vanilla extract. If you are using frozen fruit, let thaw before processing or unfreeze a bit in microwave. Blend until a creamy mixture forms.
5. Pour the filling over the crust and smooth out with spatula. Sprinkle shredded coconut for decoration.
6. Chill in the fridge overnight or place in freezer to set for at least 2–3 hours. Remove from freezer at least 1 hour before serving. Store covered in fridge for up to 4 days or freeze for up to 3 months.

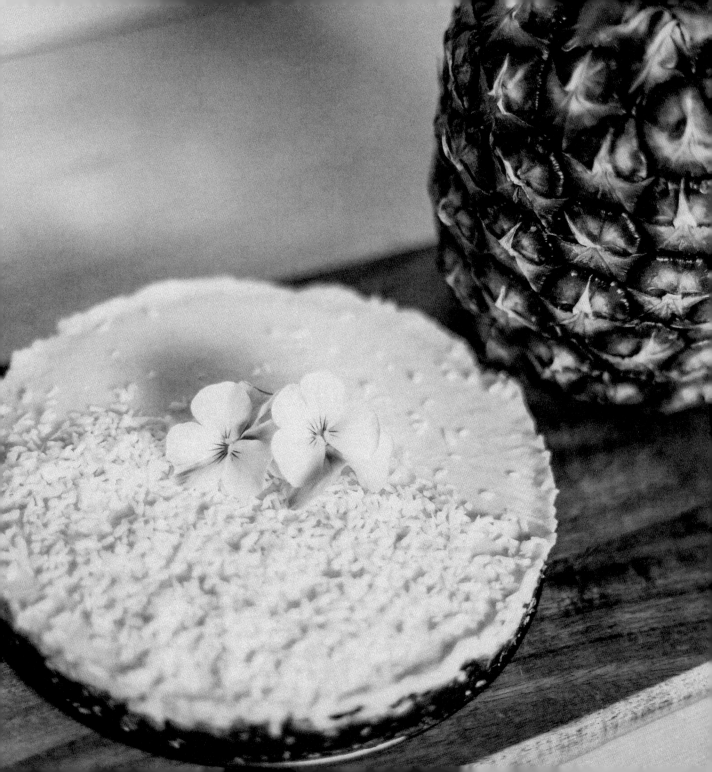

Crustless Mixed Berry Cheesecake

Sugar-free, Gluten-free, Nut-free

As you probably figured out by now, I love simple and fast recipes (ain't no time to fool around in the kitchen with three little kids!). It will take you less than 5 minutes to prepare this crustless cheesecake. If you don't believe me, time it!

Ingredients

- 1 cup cream cheese (or traditional Italian mascarpone)
- 1/4 cup heavy cream (can be omitted)
- 2 eggs
- 1 teaspoon vanilla extract
- Pinch of salt
- 2 cups mixed berries (fresh or frozen)

Directions

1. 1. Use "broil" on your oven. Preheat to 440°F/220°C.
2. In a mixing bowl, mix cream cheese, heavy cream, eggs, vanilla and salt until fully combined. I used an electric mixer to make it go faster. Gently stir in fruit. Pour the mixture into a medium round baking pan.
3. Broil for 15-20 minutes, until the cake looks firm and the top is nice and golden.
4. If desired, drizzle maple syrup on top when serving. Store in fridge for up to 3 days.

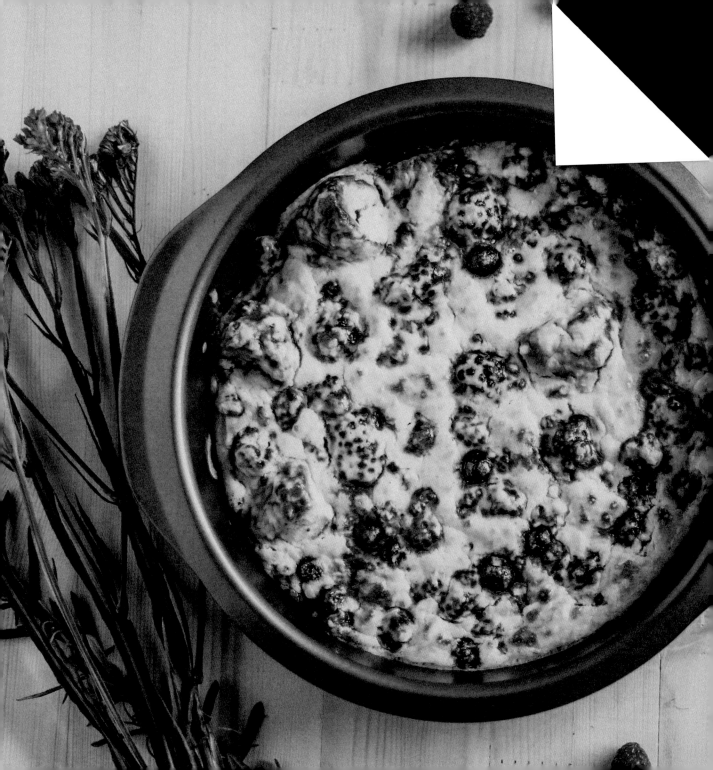

Peach Crumble

Sugar-free, Gluten-free, Dairy-free, Vegan

The smell of ripe peaches reminds me of summer! If you have some peaches that are getting too ripe and you don't have time to do anything with them, just freeze them (pitted) and have them ready for this recipe! This peach crumble is best served with homemade ice cream—a heavenly combination of a warm pie and slowly melting ice cream. Check out the "Nice Cream" section of the cookbook for recipe (page 128).

Ingredients

- 1 cup walnuts
- 1 cup oats (certified gluten-free, as needed)
- 1/2 cup butter or coconut oil for vegan version

- 1 teaspoon vanilla
- Pinch of salt
- 3 cups frozen peaches or 4-5 large ripe peaches

Directions

1. Preheat the oven to 350°F/180°C and line a square baking pan with parchment paper or use four small individual baking dishes.
2. Place walnuts into a food processor and pulse briefly to cut into smaller chunks, or skip this step if you are using crushed nuts. Stir in oats, butter or firm coconut oil, vanilla and salt. I usually use my hands to combine into a crumble.
3. Dice the peaches into bite-sized pieces and place into the baking pan. Evenly scatter the crumble over the peaches.
4. Bake for around 30 minutes, until the peach juice is bubbling around the edges of the pan and the topping is golden brown. Serve immediately, preferably with homemade ice cream. Peach crumble can be stored covered in fridge for up to 4 days.

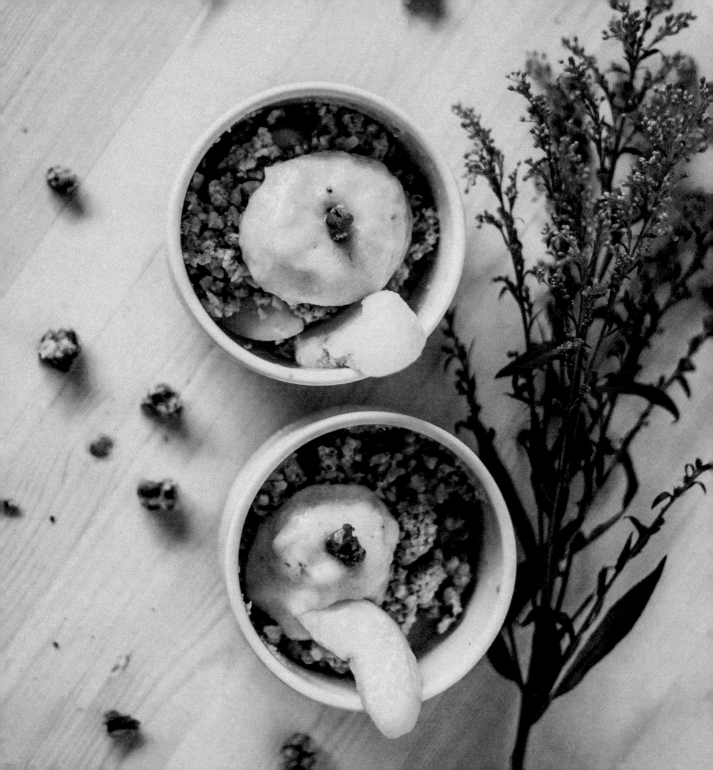

Fall Apple "Pie"

Sugar-free, Gluten-free, Dairy-free, Vegan

This is our favorite fall recipe for using our apples from our apple tree! The smell of the apples mingling with the spices is almost as rewarding as eating the pie. We love to serve it with homemade unsweetened whipped cream.

Ingredients

- 1/2 cup butter or coconut oil for vegan version
- 2 teaspoons cinnamon
- 1 teaspoon allspice
- 1 teaspoon nutmeg
- 5 apples
- 1 cup nuts of your choice (walnuts, pecans, cashews)

Directions

1. Preheat oven to 350°F/180°C and line a square baking pan with parchment paper (or I like to use a glass baking dish to make this recipe).
2. Mix melted butter or coconut oil and spices—cinnamon, allspice and nutmeg—in a mixing bowl.
3. Wash apples, remove the core and cut them into bigger pieces (leave the skin on as it contains nutrients you don't want to waste).
4. Place apple pieces into baking dish. Stir in nuts and the spice mixture. Stir well to make sure all flavors are combined.
5. Bake for 30-45 minutes, until the apples are soft. Stored covered in fridge for up to 5 days. I recommend warming again before serving.

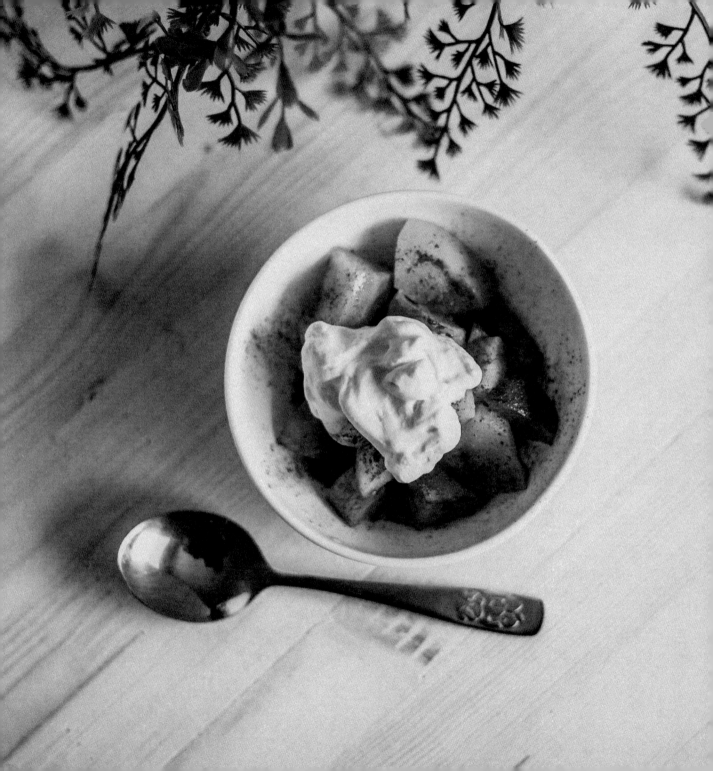

Banana Bread

Sugar-free, Gluten-free, Dairy-free, Nut-free

This banana bread is simple and fast to make. I like to serve it as a snack or even breakfast the next day. If your bananas are not very ripe, you may want to add maple syrup instead of the applesauce.

Ingredients

- 1 cup of oats (certified gluten-free, as needed)
- 3 ripe bananas (the riper the bananas, the sweeter your bread will be)
- 1/3 cup applesauce (or maple syrup)
- 1/4 cup coconut oil, melted
- 1 egg
- 1 teaspoon baking soda
- 1 teaspoon cinnamon
- Pinch of salt
- 1/2 cup raisins

Directions

1. 1. Preheat oven to 350°F/180°C. Line a rectangle bread baking tin with parchment paper (medium square tin will work well, too).
2. Blend oats in a food processor until finely ground (flour-like consistency). Add bananas, applesauce or maple syrup, melted coconut oil, egg, baking soda, cinnamon and salt and blend until well combined. Stir in raisins. Pour into baking tin.
3. Bake for around 45–50 minutes, until toothpick comes out clean (if you are using a square tin, baking time will be slightly shorter).
4. Store cooled banana bread in an airtight container at cool room temperature for 2 days, in the refrigerator for 1 week, or the freezer for up to 6 months.

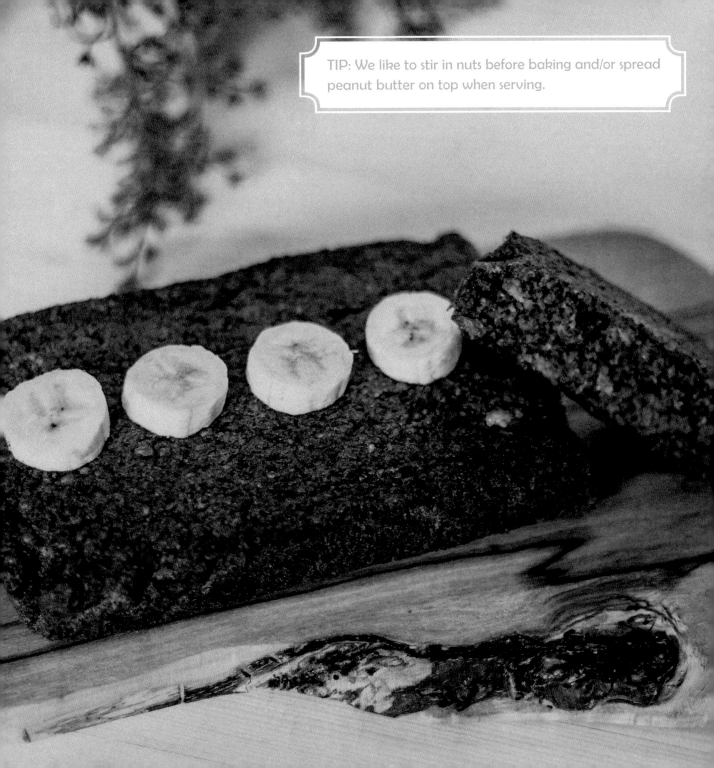

Peanut Butter Cups

Sugar-free, Gluten-free, Dairy-free, Vegan

One of my most favorite treats! I could tell you I make these for my kids, but I'm not going to lie—I LOVE peanut butter cups. Every Halloween these mysteriously go missing from my kids' treat bags, so naturally, I needed to create a recipe without sugar. Better yet, with real, whole-food ingredients. Unlike most of the recipes that you can find online, these have no added sweetener, because they are made without chocolate. Enjoy!

Ingredients

Bottom layer
- 1/2 cup dates, pitted
- 1/2 cup creamy natural peanut butter
- 2 tablespoons melted coconut oil
- 1 teaspoon vanilla extract
- 1 tablespoon raw cocoa powder

Top layer
- 1/2 cup creamy natural peanut butter
- 2 tablespoons melted coconut oil
- 1 teaspoon vanilla extract

Directions

1. Line a mini muffin tin with 24 mini-muffin baking cups.
2. Bottom layer: In a microwave-safe bowl, cover dates with water. Microwave for 1-1 1/2 minutes to soften the dates. Blend dates in a food processor until smooth. Stir in rest of the bottom-layer ingredients—peanut butter, melted coconut oil, vanilla extract and cocoa powder. Stir together well until smooth.
3. Scoop 1 teaspoon of the mixture into each mini muffin cup. If the batter is too sticky, wet the spoon. Use your fingers to gently flatten each cup. Wet your fingers with water before pressing, if needed.
4. Top layer: In a mixing bowl, stir peanut butter, melted coconut oil and vanilla extract together until smooth. Scoop 1 teaspoon of the top layer into each muffin cup. Repeat until you've filled all mini muffin cups. Then, pick up the entire muffin tin and tap and shake gently until the layer is set evenly.
5. Place muffin tin in the freezer for 30 minutes or until firm. Store in an airtight container in the freezer for up to 3 months.

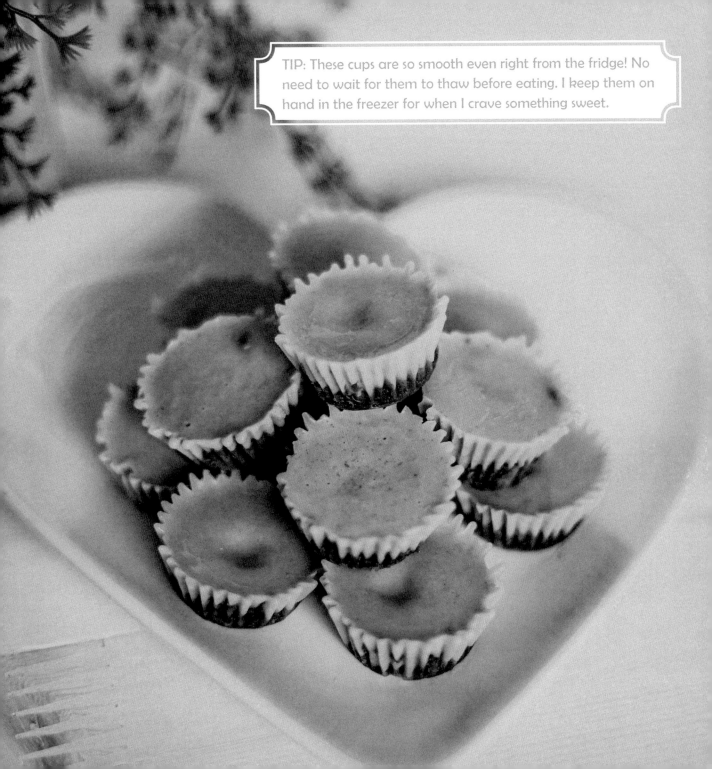

TIP: These cups are so smooth even right from the fridge! No need to wait for them to thaw before eating. I keep them on hand in the freezer for when I crave something sweet.

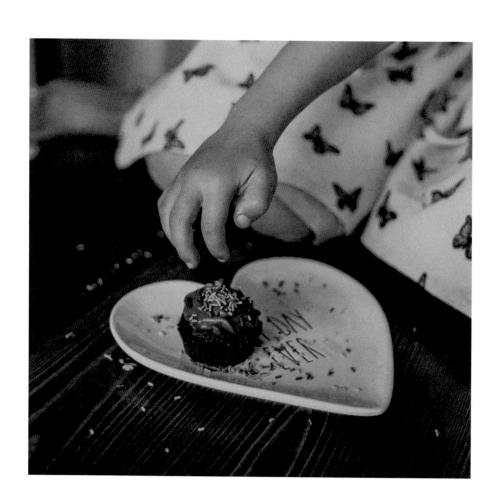

Chocolate Obsession

As I mentioned at the beginning in the recipe notes, quality dark chocolate is rich in fiber, iron, magnesium, copper, manganese and a few other minerals, but it also includes sugar. This section contains a number of recipes using chocolate chunks or chips, so they don't have the "sugar-free" label. As I strongly believe in moderation, I don't mind adding a handful of chocolate chips to a super healthy nutrition-packed recipe. You can always opt to forgo the chocolate chips, or use the darkest chocolate possible to keep the sugar content low.

This section also includes a number of chocolate recipes that don't have actual chocolate in them. They are made with raw 100% cocoa powder and sweetened with fruit. Try the Brownie Bites or Healthy Fudge and I promise, no one will ever guess they are sugar-free!

Simple Delicious Chocolate Cake

Gluten-free, Nut-free

This cake is my favorite to make for any special occasion. It looks fancy enough as a birthday cake, yet it's so simple to make! I can't be bothered to make anything that has too many steps to follow, so this cake is perfect in every way. Plus it is so chocolaty it will satisfy every chocoholic out there!

Ingredients

Cake:
- 2 cups oats (certified gluten-free, as needed)
- 3 eggs
- 1/2 cup natural plain yogurt
- 1/4 cup melted butter (can substitute with coconut oil)
- 2 ripe bananas
- 3 tablespoons raw cocoa powder
- 1 teaspoon baking soda
- 1 teaspoon vanilla extract
- Pinch of salt

Filling:
- Berry Chia Jam (see page 36)

Top Layer:
- 1 cup dairy-free chocolate (or chocolate chips of your choice)
- 1/4 cup melted butter (or coconut oil)
- Fruit of your choice for decoration

Directions

1. Preheat oven to 350°F/180°C. Line a medium round cake baking pan with parchment paper or grease with coconut oil.
2. Blend oats in a food processor until finely ground (flour-like consistency). Add remaining ingredients in the food processor, and blend until everything is evenly combined and a smooth batter forms.
3. Bake for 35–40 minutes, until toothpick comes out clean. Allow to cool.
4. When the cake is cooled down, spread a nice thick layer of jam on top of cake with the back of a spoon or spatula. Or you can cut the cake in half horizontally and spread the jam in the middle to make the cake extra moist.
5. Melt chocolate with butter or coconut oil; stir well and pour on top of the jam layer. Decorate with fruit and refrigerate for at least 2 hours, until chocolate layer is firm. Refrigerate for up to 4 days or freeze for up to 3 months.

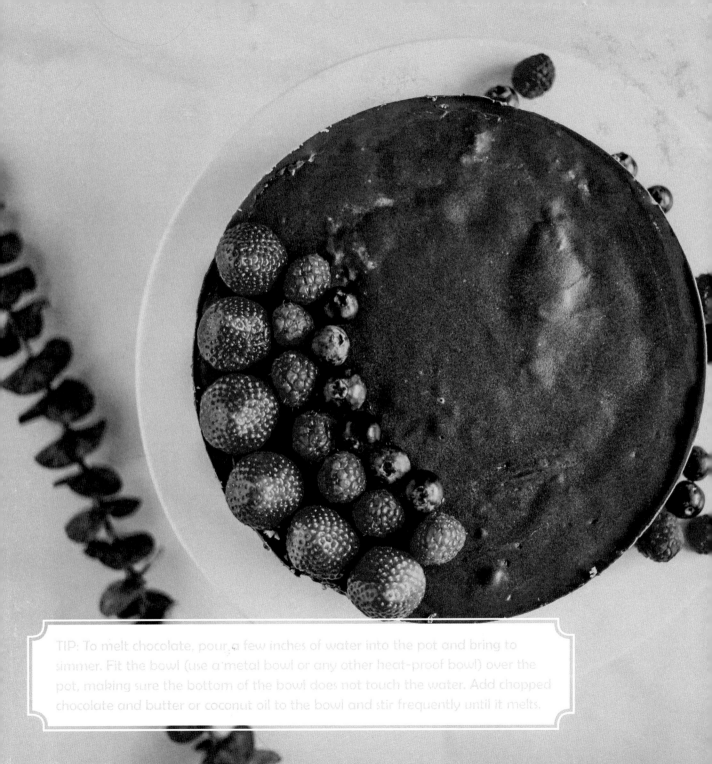

TIP: To melt chocolate, pour a few inches of water into the pot and bring to simmer. Fit the bowl (use a metal bowl or any other heat-proof bowl) over the pot, making sure the bottom of the bowl does not touch the water. Add chopped chocolate and butter or coconut oil to the bowl and stir frequently until it melts.

Chocolate Cupcakes

Gluten-free, Dairy-free, Nut-free

These look and taste almost like regular cupcakes, but they are healthy! Who says you can't have it all? Add more chocolate chips into the batter to make these cupcakes sweeter, or use dark chocolate for the icing to make them even healthier.

Ingredients

Cupcakes:
- 1 cup oats (certified gluten-free, as needed)
- 2 eggs
- 1 ripe banana
- 1/4 cup coconut oil, melted
- 2 tablespoons raw cocoa powder
- 1/2 teaspoon baking soda
- 1 teaspoon vanilla extract
- Pinch of salt

Icing:
- 1/2 cup dairy-free chocolate (or chocolate chips of your choice)
- 1 ripe banana
- 1/2 cup cream cheese (or coconut cream for dairy-free version)

Directions

1. Preheat oven to 350°F/180°C and line muffin tin with baking cups.
2. Blend oats in a food processor until finely ground (flour-like consistency). Add remaining ingredients in food processor and blend until everything is evenly combined and smooth batter forms.
3. Pour the batter into muffin cups. Bake for 20 minutes, until toothpick comes out clean. Allow to cool.
4. While the cupcakes are cooling down, melt chocolate in a microwave, double broiler or on stove top. Blend banana with cream cheese or coconut cream in a food processor. Add melted chocolate and mix together until everything is combined and creamy icing is created.
5. Frost the cupcakes. Refrigerate for at least 30 minutes before serving. Store in airtight container in fridge for up to 5 days or in freezer for up to 3 months.

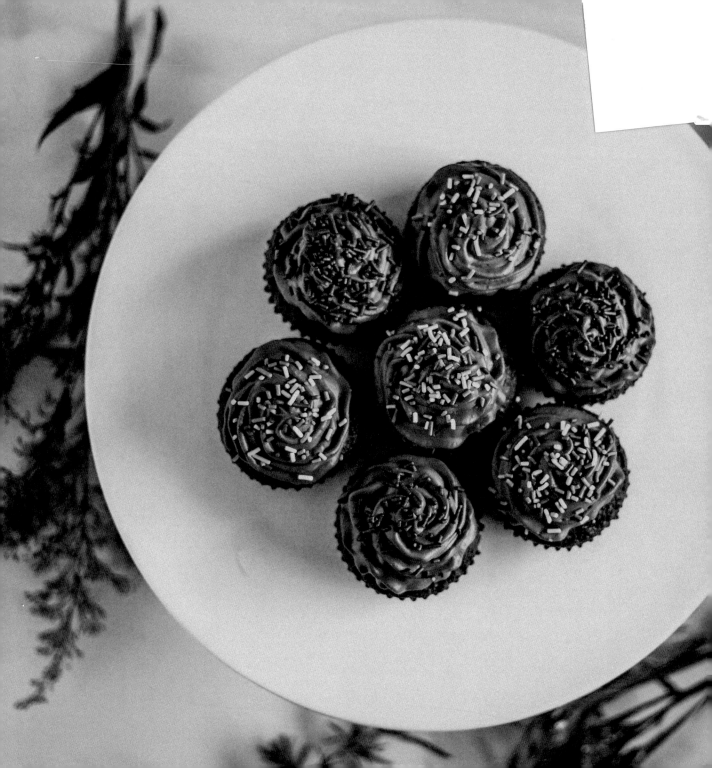

Decadent Brownie Bites

Sugar-free, Gluten-free, Dairy-free, Vegan

This recipe is loved by everyone! I definitely recommend trying it. It is gluten-free, vegan and doesn't use any sugar! The recipe calls for balsamic vinegar for a hint of flavor. I love using balsamic vinegar on green salad, but it is equally good for baking!

Ingredients

- 1 cup dates, pitted
- 1/2 cup natural almond butter (or nut butter of choice)
- 1 tablespoon flaxseed, ground
- 3 tablespoons cocoa powder

- 1/2 teaspoon baking soda
- 1 teaspoons vanilla extract
- 2 teaspoons balsamic vinegar
- Pinch of salt

Directions

1. Preheat the oven to 350°F/180°C and line a 24 mini-muffin pan with foil baking cups.
2. In a microwave-safe bowl, cover dates with water. Microwave for 1–1 1/2 minutes to soften the dates. Keep the water aside as you will use it later.
3. Blend softened dates in a food processor until smooth. Add in the almond butter, ground flaxseeds, cocoa powder, baking soda, vanilla, vinegar and 3 tablespoons of water from dates, and process again until a sticky dough is created. If the batter is too thick, add a little more water to help it blend smoothly. The mixture should still be thick and sticky, but you need to be able to combine all the ingredients together.
4. Use 1 tablespoon to scoop the dough into the mini-muffin tin. Water the spoon after each scoop to prevent sticking. Use your wet fingers to gently flatten each mini muffin. Wet your fingers before pressing so they won't stick to the batter.
5. Bake for 12–15 minutes. The centers will still feel slightly soft to the touch, but the top should look firm. Let the brownies cool completely, at least 30 minutes. They are very soft and fragile and may be difficult to remove from pan.

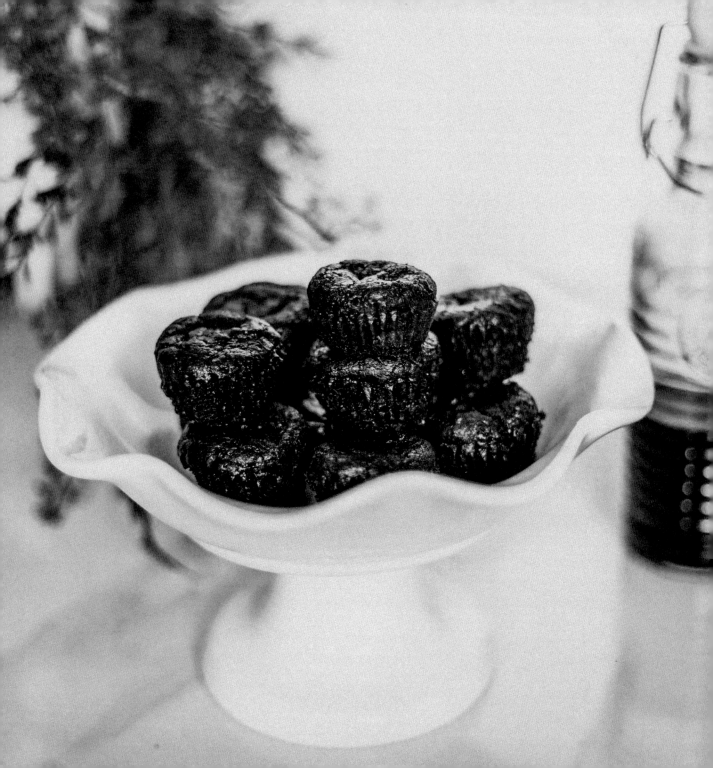

Black Bean Brownies

Gluten-free, Dairy-free, Vegan, Nut-free

These brownies are so good, no one will ever believe they are made from beans instead of flour. Don't tell anyone what is in them and I bet you will get so many compliments. They are soft, sweet and SO good!

Ingredients

- 1/2 cup oats (certified gluten-free, as needed)
- 1 1/2 cup black beans, rinsed
- 1 banana
- 1/2 cup coconut oil
- 2 tablespoons cocoa powder
- 1 teaspoon pure vanilla extract
- 1/2 teaspoon baking soda
- Pinch of salt
- 1/2 cup dairy-free chocolate (or chocolate chips of your choice)

Directions

1. Preheat oven to 350°F/180°C. Line a small square baking pan with parchment paper.
2. Blend oats in a food processor until finely ground (flour-like consistency). Add remaining ingredients, except for chocolate chips, in food processor and blend until smooth.
3. Stir in the chocolate chips. Pour batter into baking pan.
4. Bake for 20-25 minutes. The centers will still feel slightly soft to the touch, but the top should look firm. Allow brownies to completely cool (at least 15 minutes) before cutting and serving.

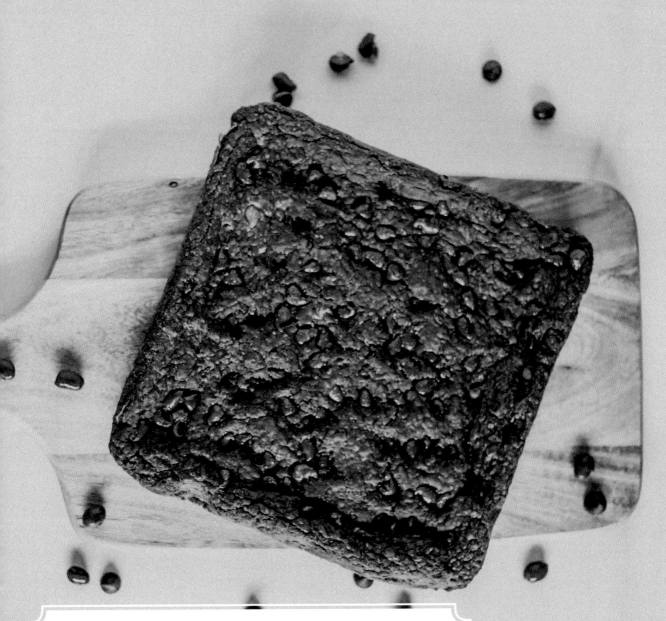

TIP: If the brownies are too soft or crumbly when trying to cut them, put them in the fridge for a couple of hours and they will firm up. Store in a covered, airtight container and refrigerate for up to 5 days or freeze for up to 3 months.

Zucchini Brownies

Gluten-free, Dairy-free

Let's talk about zucchini. It is a perfect summer vegetable and very easy to grow. Every summer, I get at least one person asking me, "What should I do with all my zucchini?" Our family likes to marinade zucchini in olive oil, salt and garlic, and BBQ it on the grill as a side dish. I also really like to cut zucchini with a spiralizer to make spaghetti or for adding to scrambled eggs. But brownies are always a great idea . . . right?!

Ingredients

- 1 cup finely shredded zucchini
- 1/2 cup natural almond butter (or nut/ seed butter of choice)
- 1 ripe banana
- 1 large egg
- 1/4 cup raw cocoa powder

- 1 tablespoon maple syrup (optional)
- 1 teaspoon vanilla
- 1/2 teaspoon baking soda
- Pinch of salt
- 1/2 cup dairy-free chocolate (or chocolate chips of your choice)

Directions

1. Preheat oven to 350°F/180°C. Line small square baking pan with parchment paper.
2. Shred zucchini using the small holes on the grater to get very thin shreds. Squeeze all the moisture out and set aside.
3. In a food processor, blend almond butter, banana, egg, cocoa powder, maple syrup, vanilla and baking soda until everything is evenly combined.
4. Stir in the zucchini until batter is evenly mixed. Gently stir in chocolate chips. Pour batter into prepared pan.
5. Bake in the oven for about 30 minutes or until toothpick comes out clean. Allow brownies to cool before cutting and serving.

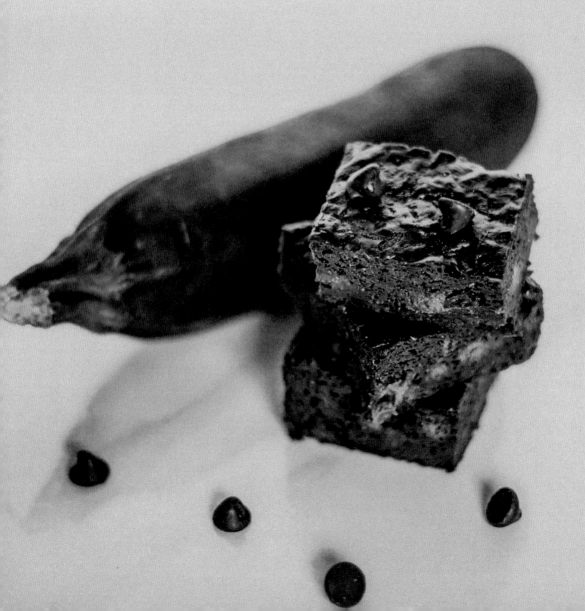

TIP: Eat these brownies the next day from the fridge and the flavor and sweetness come out even more! Store in a covered, airtight container and refrigerate for up to 5 days or freeze for up to 3 months

Dark Chocolate Raspberry Brownies

Gluten-free, Dairy-free, Nut-free

These are my personal favorite. They are best eaten the next day from the fridge and I love to enjoy them with my coffee. This recipe is super-fast to make and contains ingredients I always have on hand. The combination of dark chocolate and raspberries is delicious! You may want to add maple syrup or the sweetener of your choice, as my kids don't find them sweet enough.

Ingredients

- 3 eggs
- 1/2 cup coconut oil, melted
- 1/4 cup raw cocoa powder
- 1 teaspoon vanilla
- Pinch of sea salt
- 1/2 cup 70% dark chocolate chunks
- 1 cup raspberries (fresh or frozen)

Directions

1. Preheat oven to 400°F/200°C. Line medium square baking pan with parchment paper.
2. Whisk eggs in a mixing bowl (by hand or with electric mixer). Add melted coconut oil, cocoa, vanilla and salt, and mix until combined and smooth batter forms.
3. Gently stir through raspberries and chocolate chunks. Pour batter into pan and level out with spatula.
4. Bake for 25 minutes. Brownies will still look soft, but will firm up when they cool down. Let cool in fridge for at least an hour before serving. Store in a covered airtight container and refrigerate for up to 5 days or freeze for up to 3 months.

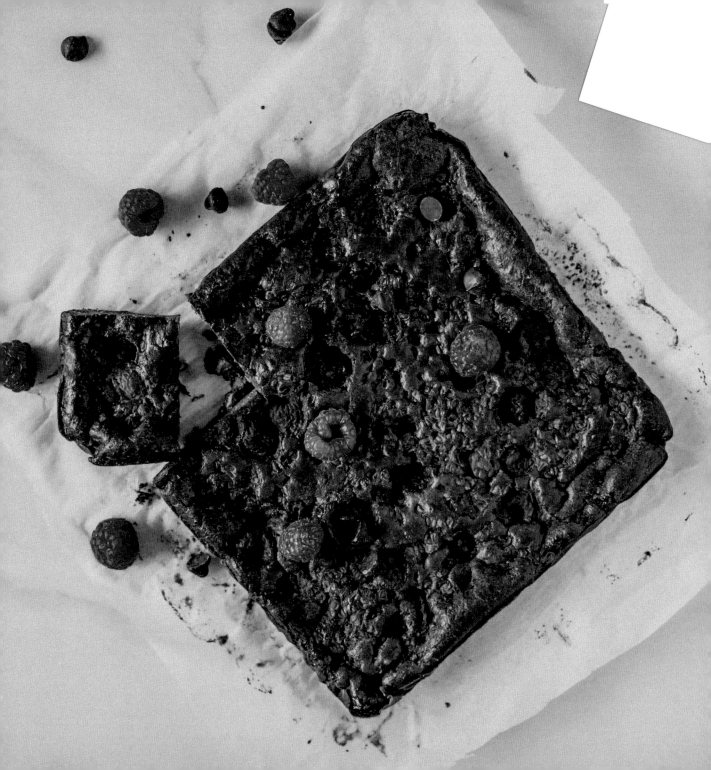

Healthy Fudge

Sugar-free, Gluten-free, Dairy-free, Vegan, Nut-free

This is another recipe I have from the amazing health warrior, Dr. Lindsay Gee (check out the Mighty Muffin recipe on page 42 to read more about Lindsay). I love to have this recipe on hand when that sweet tooth comes for an (uninvited) visit. Seriously a must-try recipe and my husband Andy's favorite!

Ingredients

- 1 cup dates, pitted
- 1 ripened banana
- 1 teaspoon vanilla extract (or mint extract)
- 1/2 cup coconut oil
- 2/3 cup cocoa powder
- Nuts or dried fruit of your liking (optional)

Directions

1. Soften dates by putting them in a microwave-safe bowl, covering them with water and microwaving them for 1 1/2 minutes.
2. Throw the softened dates and ripened banana in a food processor and blend until smooth. Add melted coconut oil, cocoa powder, vanilla or mint extract, and salt, and process until everything comes together in a smooth mixture.
3. Add any nuts or dried fruit you like or omit to keep pure "chocolate" version. Place the fudge in the fridge or freezer until it firms up before serving.

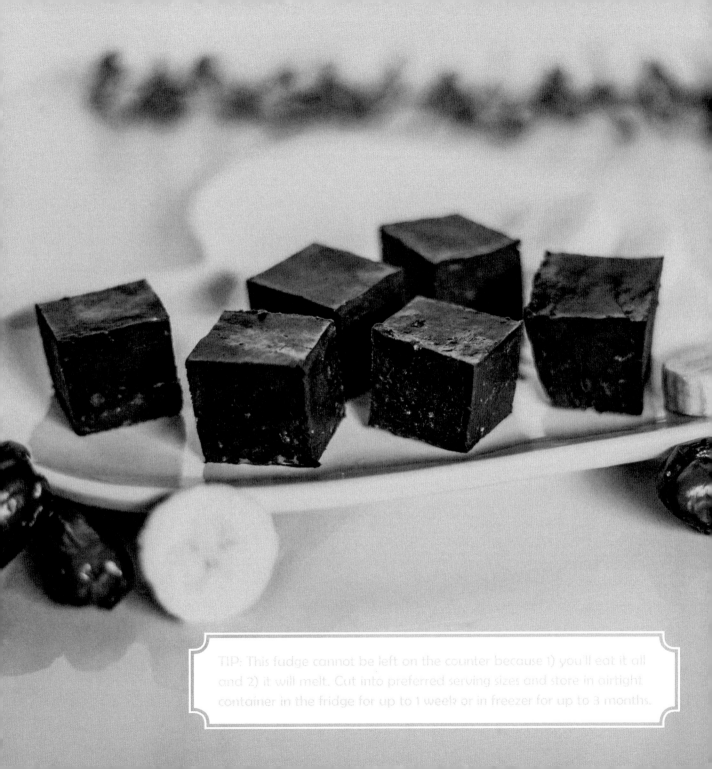

Chocolate Pudding

Sugar-free, Gluten-free, Dairy-free, Vegan, Nut-free

I purposely didn't call this recipe avocado pudding, because I know the combination of avocado and chocolate is not appealing to everyone. But I encourage you to put your prejudices aside and try it! This is a simple way of making a chocolate pudding without sugar or dairy.

Ingredients

- 1/2 cup dates
- 2 ripe bananas
- 1 ripe avocado
- 3 teaspoons raw cocoa powder

Directions

1. Soften dates by putting them in a bowl, covering them with water, then microwaving them for 1 minute. Strain the water.
2. Blend the softened dates in a food processor.
3. Add the bananas, avocado and cocoa powder and blend until everything is smooth and nicely combined.
4. Place into small bowls and serve immediately.

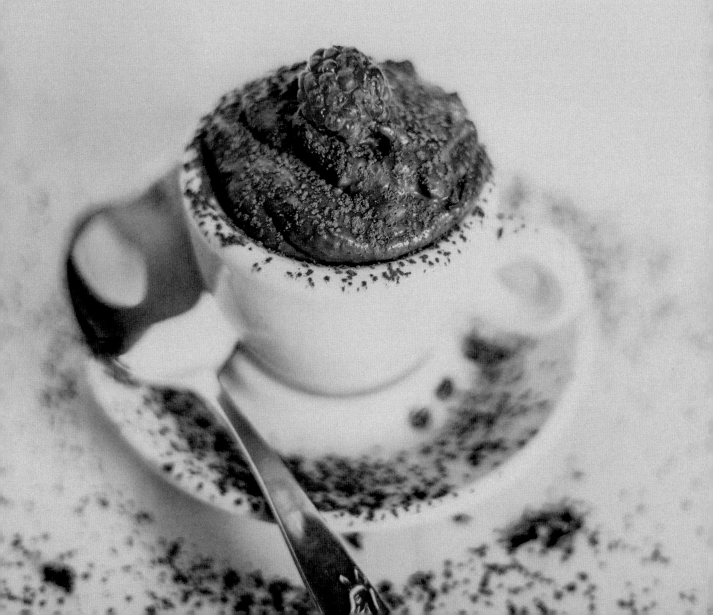

TIP: You can add fresh fruit like strawberries or raspberries when serving the pudding. If your bananas are not very ripe, add a little bit of maple syrup.

Vegan Chocolate Cheesecake Cups

Gluten-free, Dairy-free, Vegan

This recipe was created when I had extra homemade granola on hand and was trying to quickly come up with a fancy dessert that didn't require baking. It gets bonus points for being plant-based and gluten-free. You're welcome!

Ingredients (to make 4 small cups)

- 1 banana
- 1 cup coconut cream
- 1/2 cup dairy-free chocolate
- 1 cup Homemade Granola (see recipe on page 28)
- 1 cup fresh or frozen strawberries

Directions

1. Melt chocolate in a double boiler, in a microwave or on stove top.
2. In a food processor, mix banana and coconut cream until combined. Add the melted chocolate and process until everything comes together into a nice, smooth chocolate cream.
3. Layer the cups with 1/4 cup of granola on bottom of each cup. Add 1/4 cup of strawberries and top with chocolate cream.
4. Refrigerate for 2-3 hours before serving. Store covered in refrigerator for up to 4 days.

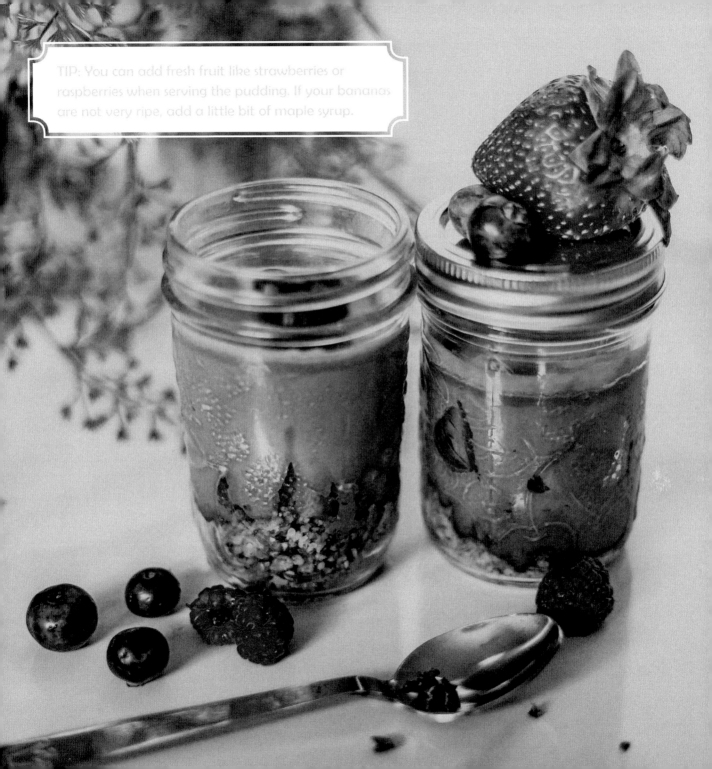

TIP: You can add fresh fruit like strawberries or raspberries when serving the pudding. If your bananas are not very ripe, add a little bit of maple syrup.

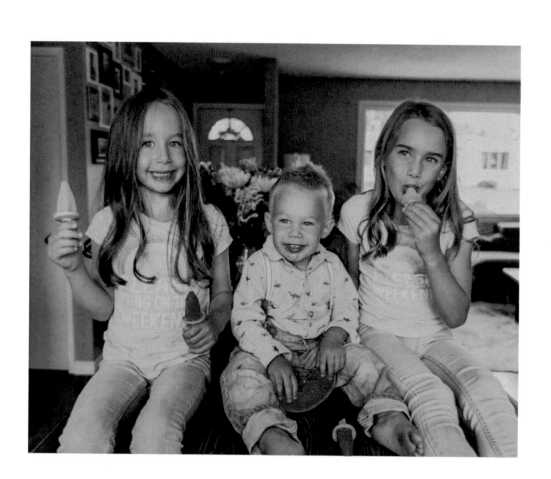

(N)Ice Cream & Popsicles

Everyone screams for ice cream, especially on a hot summer day. So, what is our healthy alternative to have on hand at home? Let me introduce you, if you haven't met already, to nice cream and popsicles (ice pops)! Nice cream is basically a bunch of frozen fruit with or without a splash of milk of your choice or coconut cream, blended into an "ice cream" form to be enjoyed immediately. Popsicles are like smoothies, but put into a fun mold to be frozen before eating. Most store-bought popsicles' main ingredient is—you guessed it—sugar. Some of the popsicles are made with 100% juice, but as I mentioned at the beginning of my book, this juice is just fruit sugar without the fiber and other nutrients. By blending your own fruit, you are keeping all the nutrients. These will take you less than 5 minutes to make and your kids will love them! Buy some fun molds online and you will be winning this summer. You can mix and match your flavors—or, better yet, let your kids to make their own nice cream or popsicles by using the ingredients in your freezer and their imagination. My kids love to make them as much as they enjoy eating them!

Popsicles

Sugar-free, Gluten-free, Dairy-free, Vegan, Nut-free, Raw

You can mix and match your flavors of choice, but here are some of our favorite combinations. I recommend buying silicon molds so the popsicles are easier to remove.

Summer (Watermelon & Strawberry) Popsicles

Ingredients

- 1 cup watermelon
- 1 cup strawberries
- 1 teaspoon lemon juice

Tropical (Mango, Pineapple & Coconut) Popsicles

Ingredients

- 1 cup pineapple
- 1 cup mango
- 1/2 cup coconut milk or cream

Blueberry Cream Popsicles

Ingredients

- 1 1/2 cup blueberries
- 1/2 cup natural plain yogurt (or milk of your choice)
- 1 teaspoon lemon juice
- 1 teaspoon vanilla extract
- 1 teaspoon maple syrup (optional)

Directions

1. Pulse all ingredients together in a blender until smooth.
2. Pour into popsicle molds and freeze until firm.

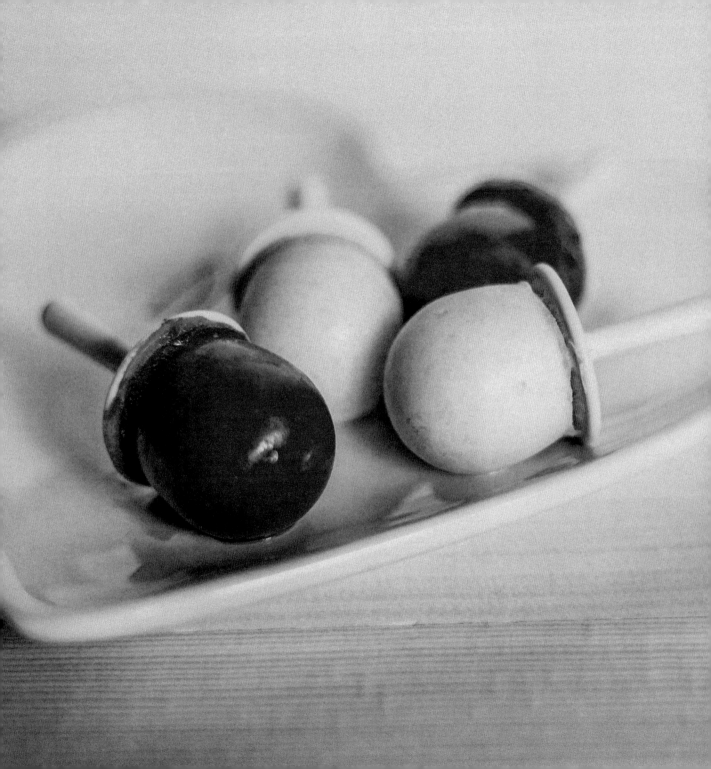

Banana Nice Cream with Add-ins

Sugar-free, Gluten-free, Dairy-free, Vegan, Nut-free, Raw

This is the basic banana nice cream recipe that serves as a base. You can mix and match any flavors you like; below are some of our favorite combinations. I usually have frozen banana slices on hand in our freezer. This is a great way to use your bananas that are getting too ripe.

Ingredients

- 1 large banana
- 2 tablespoons unsweetened almond milk (or milk of your choice)

Directions

1. Peel and slice banana and place in freezer for at least a couple of hours or up to 3 months.
2. When ready to make nice cream: Blend frozen banana slices and almond milk in food processor until smooth. Scrape the sides and mix some more. Add more milk if needed.
3. Serve immediately for "soft-serve" consistency or transfer into freezer-friendly container and freeze for 2 hours. Stir occasionally. If you freeze it for longer (or overnight), you will need to take it out 15-30 minutes before serving to be able to scoop it out.

Add-ins:

Peanut Butter - Add 1 tablespoon peanut butter into food processor when mixing

Chocolate - Add 2 tablespoons of raw cocoa powder into food processor when mixing and stir in 1/4 cup of mini chocolate chips before serving

Strawberries - Add 1/2 cup strawberries (fresh or frozen)

Mint Chip - Replace the almond milk with 1/4 cup coconut cream and add 1/4 teaspoon mint extract. Stir in 1/4 cup mini chocolate chips before serving. For "minty" color, add pinch of spirulina or natural food coloring.

Peach - Add 1/2 cup peaches (fresh or frozen)

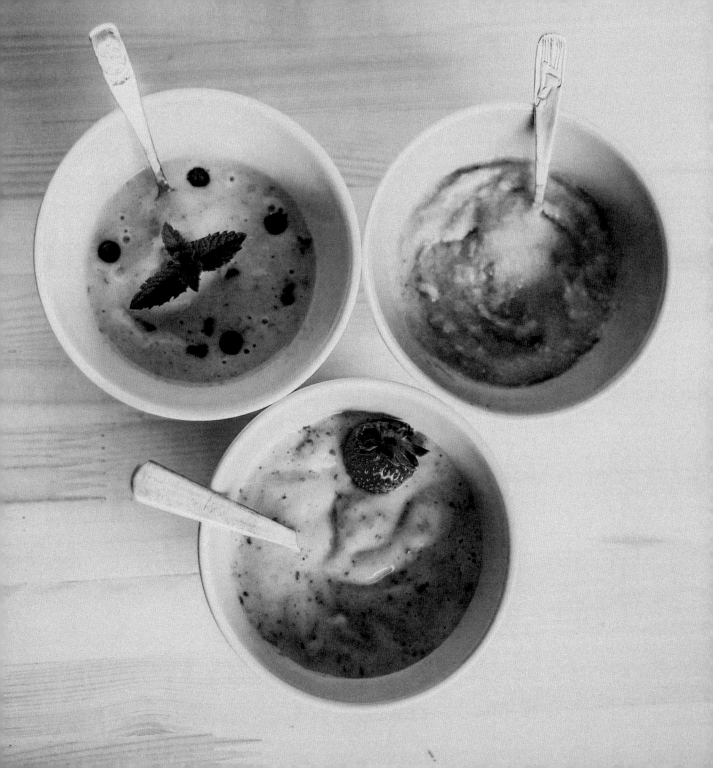

Cherry Chocolate Ice Cream

Gluten-free, Dairy-free, Vegan, Nut-free, Raw

My ALL TIME favorite ice cream! I hope you love it as much as I do. Enjoy, you deserve it mama!

Ingredients

- Coconut cream from one can—approximately 1 cup of coconut cream (see page 15 for how to get coconut cream)
- 1 cup strawberries (fresh or frozen)
- 1 cup cherries, pitted (fresh or frozen), **divided use**
- 1/2 cup dark chocolate chunks

Directions

1. In food processor, mix coconut cream, strawberries and 1/2 cup of cherries until everything is combined and smooth. You may need to scrape the sides of the food processor a few times.
2. Stir in (don't blend) the second 1/2 cup of cherries, cut into smaller pieces, and the dark chocolate chunks.
3. If you used frozen fruit, you may enjoy your ice cream immediately as a soft serve, or put into freezer-friendly container and freeze for 2-3 hours. Stir occasionally so it freezes evenly (I always forget this step!). If it's too hard, let thaw for 15-30 minutes before serving.

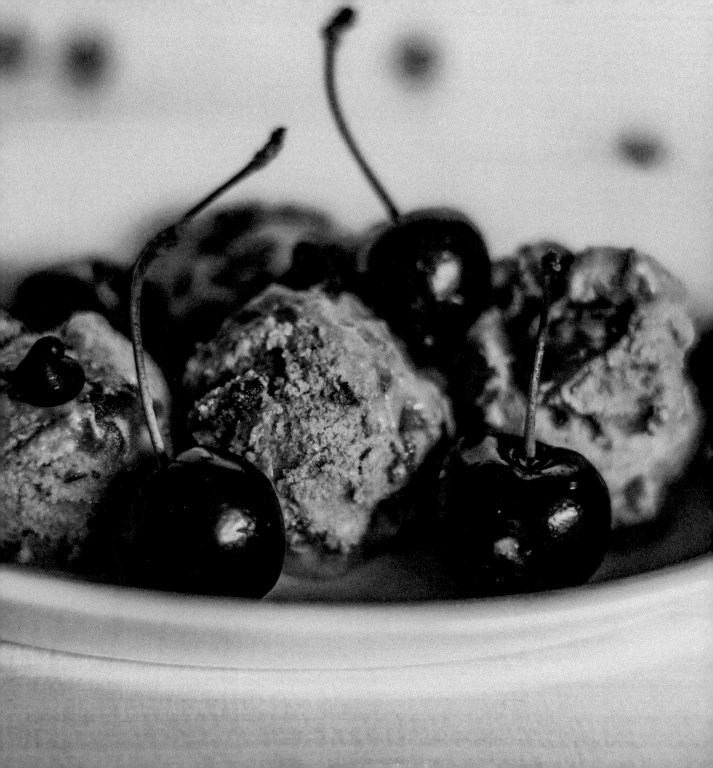

Acknowledgments

As much as I always loved to write and considered studying journalism after I graduated, writing in English was definitely a big challenge for me. I would love to mention a few special people who helped me to make my dream (this cookbook) a reality.

First of all, thanks to my husband for supporting me when I came up with the crazy idea to actually put all my sugar-free treats on paper and publish them. Huge thanks to my "mama bear" squad, all the talented strong moms I'm fortunate to have in my life who helped me bring this book to life! A special mention to Ashley Despres with Ash of All Arts, the most talented and creative photographer (amongst her many other skills). When I decided to make this cookbook, I knew right away she would be the one taking the pictures. Thank you, Ashley, for capturing my recipes on point with your creative touch! Special thanks to Andrea Adams for editing the book and providing feedback, making my cookbook the best it could be! Andrea is a busy mom with three little kids and a successful career, and she still manages to be fit, healthy and fabulous— exactly my book audience! Thanks to another super successful mama bear, Rowena Cui, owner of PlanIT Sound, the marketing wizard who is helping me spread awareness and bring my sugar-free treats cookbook to all the busy moms out there! To my bestie Srnka—thanks for testing all the treats and coming up with the idea for the title. And the rest of my squad—Dana, Amanda, Kendra, Kobi, Kassandra, Randi, Kim, Candace, Heather, Camilla, Kika, Janka and Baja—thanks for your unconditional support! This motherhood thing is definitely easier when you have your girlfriends around! Thanks to my sisters, Neta and Sandra, for cheering me on from far away.

And lastly, thanks to my mom for watching over me since the day I lost her! There is so much good in my life and I know it's thanks to her!

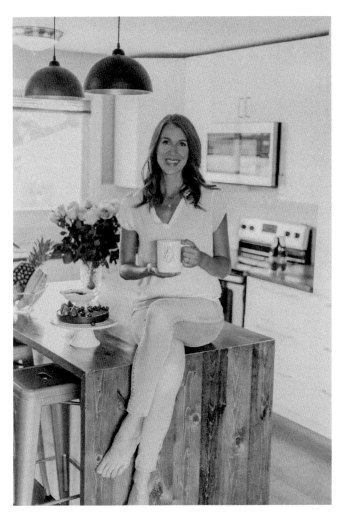

Nela Kovacovic is a mom of three littles—Ariana, Arwen and Alex. She is originally from the small European country of Slovakia, living her American dream in Canada. She is an international award-winning event planner, with experience producing live shows in Europe and Canada. When the world pandemic hit and all events were canceled, she finally had time to pursue her passion and put on paper all her famous sugar-free treat recipes.

Nela believes in the power of cooking and baking with kids, sharing nutritional knowledge from a young age. She is an advocate for fit families and her mission is to bring awareness to how we can all make small adjustments in life to raise a generation of healthy and strong kids!

IG: @sugarfreetreatsforkids

Website: www.sugarfreetreatsforkids.com

Manufactured by Amazon.ca
Bolton, ON

21465876R00086